DIABETES

Skyhorse Publishing books may be purchased in bulk at special discounts for sales promotion, corporate gifts, fund-raising, or educational purposes. Special editions can also be created to specifications. For details, contact the Special Sales Department, Skyhorse Publishing, 555 Eighth Avenue, Suite 903, New York, NY 10018 or info@skyhorsepublishing.com.

www.skyhorsepublishing.com

10 9 8 7 6 5 4 3 2 1

Library of Congress Cataloging-in-Publication Data

Kingham, Karen.
 Eat well live well with diabetes : low-GI recipes and tips / by Karen Kingham.
   p. cm.
 Includes index.
 ISBN 978-1-60239-672-2
 1. Diabetes–Diet therapy–Recipes. 2. Glycemic index. I. Title.
 RC662.K56 2009
 616.4'62–dc22
                              2009019440

Printed in China

IMPORTANT: Those who might be at risk from the effects of salmonella poisoning (the elderly, pregnant women, young children and those suffering from immune deficiency diseases) should consult their doctor with any concerns about eating raw eggs.

NOTE: You may find cooking times vary depending on the oven you are using. For convection ovens, as a general rule, set the oven temperature to 35°F lower than indicated in the recipe.

EATWELLLIVEWELL
with
DIABETES
Low-GI recipes and tips

Introductory text by Karen Kingham (nutritionist)

Skyhorse Publishing

CONTENTS

LIVING WITH DIABETES

Diabetes affects more than 230 million people worldwide and is one of the fastest growing diseases in the world. Because the risk of developing diabetes is influenced by lifestyle, there are steps you can take to reduce this risk, control it once you've been diagnosed or even reverse some of its unwanted effects.

In the past, people with diabetes followed rigid diet plans with little room for enjoyment. Today, thanks to good scientific research, diet and lifestyle recommendations for diabetes differ very little from those made for everyone else: a healthy diet balanced for your individual needs, plus daily exercise.

You may also be pleasantly surprised to learn that healthy food can be, and is, delicious if you know how to prepare it. And, once you get to the end of this book, you will be convinced of it.

Who will benefit from this book?

If you have diabetes or are at risk of developing it, or you care for someone who has it, then you will find this book useful. Diabetes doesn't have to mean separate meals or eating differently than everyone else. All the recipes in this book can be enjoyed by family and friends alike, which is especially important when children have diabetes. No child wants to be different, and in many ways their diet doesn't have to be. The recipes in this book will help them—or anyone else for that matter—achieve a healthy, balanced diet.

What is diabetes?

Diabetes results in a buildup of sugar (known as glucose) in the bloodstream. This happens when the body can't make enough of the hormone insulin, or is unable to use insulin properly.

To understand why and how this happens you need to understand a little about how the body works. The level of glucose in the blood rises whenever you eat any carbohydrate (sugars or starches). As the carbohydrate is digested, glucose is absorbed into the bloodstream. As the blood glucose level rises, it stimulates the pancreas to release the hormone insulin. The insulin enables the body's cells to absorb the glucose from the blood so that the cells can use it for energy (or store it to use as energy later on).

Insulin works much like a key, fitting into a lock that opens the cell's door. Without insulin, glucose remains trapped within the blood. The action of insulin, in concert with other hormones, keeps you blood glucose level steady.

Diabetes develops when the pancreas either doesn't make enough insulin or the body becomes resistant to the effects of insulin. In both cases, the result is that glucose is unable to get to the cells and builds up in the bloodstream.

Over time, a high blood glucose level can damage the eyes, nerves and blood vessels as well as increase the risk of heart disease, kidney and circulation problems. Early diagnosis and good blood glucose control are essential in preventing these serious health problems.

There are several different types of diabetes and they all result in too much glucose in the bloodstream:

Type 1 diabetes

Sometimes called insulin-dependent diabetes or juvenile-onset diabetes, type 1 diabetes is the least common but the most serious form of diabetes. It typically begins in childhood or early adulthood but can occur at any age.

Type 1 diabetes is an autoimmune disease in which the body's immune system destroys cells in the pancreas that are responsible for making insulin. Scientists believe that exposure to a particular virus or chemical may trigger this immune reaction in susceptible people.

Ultimately, the pancreas stops making insulin and the blood glucose level rises dramatically. The symptoms that result include excessive thirst, frequent urination, blurred vision, abdominal cramps and nausea.

Weight loss is also very common as the body burns up fat and muscle tissue to use as energy instead of blood glucose. Symptoms will usually appear very suddenly due to the speed in which glucose builds up in the blood once insulin production fails.

Unlike the other forms of diabetes, excess weight is not the reason for the development of type 1 diabetes, and most people are a healthy weight at the time their diabetes begins.

Blood glucose levels in type 1 diabetes are managed with regular daily insulin injections, healthy eating and an active lifestyle.

Type 2 diabetes

Also known as non-insulin dependent diabetes or adult onset diabetes, this type of diabetes is the most common, affecting up to 90 percent of all people with diabetes.

Type 2 diabetes is largely found in people over 40 years of age who are overweight and have a family history of diabetes. However, recently, type 2 diabetes is being seen in younger adults and even children, due to our population becoming less active and more overweight.

In type 2 diabetes the pancreas continues to make insulin (unlike type 1 diabetes) but the body doesn't respond to it as well and becomes resistant to its effects. This is known as insulin resistance. The pancreas makes more insulin to compensate, but over time this still isn't enough. Eventually the blood glucose level remains elevated.

The onset of type 2 diabetes is typically a gradual process, unlike type 1 diabetes. In fact, many people with type 2 diabetes won't have any noticeable symptoms early on and so won't be aware they have the condition. Once blood glucose begins to rise significantly, the following symptoms may be experienced: excessive thirst, frequent urination, blurred vision, thrush, frequent infections, poor wound healing and fatigue.

Type 2 diabetes can often be managed with healthy eating, an active lifestyle and weight loss alone. The best way to achieve this will be different for every individual, so it is important to follow the advice of a doctor, dietitian or diabetes educator. In addition to losing weight with healthy diet and exercise, some people with type 2 diabetes might also need medication. This may be tablets that help reduce insulin resistance and, in some cases, insulin injections as well.

Risk factors for type 2 diabetes

If you have one or more of the following factors, then you are at risk for type 2 diabetes and should visit your doctor as soon as possible.

- I am over 45 years old and overweight
- I am over 45 years old and have high blood pressure
- I am over 45 years old and do very little physical activity
- I am over 45 years old and have one or more family members with diabetes
- I am over 35 years old and am of Asian, Southern European, Indian, Hispanic, Aboriginal, Torres Strait Islander or Polynesian descent
- I am over 55 years old
- I have had a heart attack or stroke
- I have had gestational diabetes or my baby weighed over 8 lb 12 oz at birth
- I am overweight and have polycystic ovarian syndrome (PCOS)
- I am overweight, with most of my weight around my middle rather than on my hips and thighs
- I have high blood pressure, a high blood cholesterol or high triglyceride level

Gestational diabetes

Gestational diabetes is a type of diabetes, usually temporary, that develops during pregnancy, around the second or third trimester. Insulin needs are higher in pregnancy and the hormones produced during this time can reduce the effectiveness of insulin. It is diagnosed by a blood test at around 24 to 28 weeks gestation and is similar to type 2 diabetes where the body is resistant to the effects of insulin.

It is estimated that between 3 and 8 percent of pregnant women can't meet their body's extra demands for insulin and end up with gestational diabetes. Women at greatest risk are those over 30 years of age with a family history of type 2 diabetes and those who are overweight. Other risk factors include being of Chinese, Indian or Aboriginal descent or previously having had a baby weighing more than 8 lb 12 oz.

Gestational diabetes is controlled with a healthy diet, an active lifestyle and strict monitoring of blood glucose levels. If this isn't enough to keep blood glucose levels in check then insulin injections are needed and some women may need to be admitted to the hospital. Well-managed blood glucose levels are important to your health and the baby's. Poorly controlled blood glucose levels cause your baby to grow bigger and fatter. This makes delivery more difficult and increases the risk of complications such as miscarriage and health problems for the baby.

Gestational diabetes usually goes away once the baby is born but it does increase the risk for developing type 2 diabetes later in life for both you and your child. These risks can be reduced by maintaining a healthy weight, eating a healthy diet and staying active.

Pre-diabetes

Pre-diabetes occurs when blood glucose levels are higher than normal but not high enough to be diagnosed as diabetes. It is also known as Impaired Glucose Tolerance (IGT) or Impaired Fasting Glucose (IFG).

Like type 2 diabetes, pre-diabetes is due to the body becoming resistant to the effects of insulin. The risk of pre-diabetes becoming type 2 diabetes is high. However, research shows that you can reverse this risk simply by improving your diet and lifestyle. This means controlling your weight, losing weight if you are carrying excess, reducing the amount of fat you eat, increasing your fiber intake, switching to low glycemic index carbohydrates and being more active—aiming for at least 30 minutes of exercise a day, or more if you need to lose weight. In fact, research shows that these strategies can be even more effective than medication in reversing the progress of pre-diabetes toward type 2 diabetes.

How common is diabetes?

The International Diabetes Federation estimates that six million people worldwide develop diabetes each year, and that in some countries as many as 80 percent of these people won't know it. They also predict that by 2025, diabetes will affect 350 million people, which is equivalent to a serious, worldwide diabetes epidemic.

Why is diabetes on the increase? The most important factor is the ever-expanding weight of the world's population. The rise in diabetes is closely coupled to rising rates of obesity. In some countries obesity rates have more than tripled in the last 20 years, and there are now around 1.3 billion overweight people in the world—which outnumbers the world's starving. It is little wonder then that the chronic illnesses brought on by obesity—like type 2 diabetes—are also on the rise.

In many ways the statistics are more alarming for those who are not yet diagnosed. Being unaware of your diabetes puts you at greater risk of health complications from chronically-high blood glucose levels. For this reason everyone at risk of diabetes (see page 10) should make it a priority to have regular checkups with their doctor.

What health problems can be caused by diabetes?

Damage to the body occurs when blood glucose levels are chronically high. Over time, this may result in permanent damage to your blood vessels and the tissues or organs they supply. In the case of type 2 diabetes this may have been happening for some time before you even know about it. In many cases, the complications of high blood glucose levels (nerve problems, heart attack, vision disturbances) lead to a diagnosis of type 2 diabetes.

Once you have been diagnosed with diabetes, keeping your blood glucose level within the normal range, or as close to the normal range as possible, is vital. By doing this you can prevent or slow the onset of the serious health complications associated with diabetes. The most common complications include:

Cardiovascular disease

People with diabetes are around five times more likely to develop heart disease and can be up to four times more likely to suffer a stroke than those without diabetes.

Damage to blood vessels caused by diabetes also affects the circulation, particularly in the legs. This poor circulation makes cuts and infections slow to heal. A diet low in saturated fat and high in fiber with antioxidant-rich vegetables and fruit is essential when you have diabetes for reducing your risk of cardiovascular desease.

Nerve damage

Also known as neuropathy, nerve damage results in the loss of sensation and/or pain in the hands and feet as well as problems with the functioning of many of the body's systems.

One of the complications of nerve damage, especially affecting the legs and feet, occurs when numbness allows injuries to go unnoticed. People with diabetes should have regular foot checkups for this reason.

Kidney disease

Kidney disease can occur when the blood vessels of the kidney are damaged by high blood glucose. Diabetes is a leading cause of kidney failure and people with diabetes are four times more likely to develop kidney disease than someone without diabetes.

Eye diseases

Diabetic retinopathy, a disease affecting the blood vessels of the retina, is the most common eye-related complication of diabetes. Keeping eye problems at bay can be helped by having regular checkups with your ophthalmologist (eye specialist) or optometrist. A diet rich in vegetables and fruits will also help as antioxidants help protect the delicate blood vessels in eyes.

Living well with diabetes

Taking control of your diabetes means having the knowledge and support to make the best choices about your health and lifestyle. Access to health professionals such as your doctor, diabetes specialist physician, dietitian, diabetes educator, podiatrist and ophthalmologist (eye specialist) will mean the changes you make will be based on accurate up-to-date medical information. It is important to follow-up with your health team regularly to make sure that your blood glucose remains sufficiently under control.

Joining your local diabetes support group will also offer enormous benefits in terms of advice, support, reduced price products and many other services.

Why change your diet and lifestyle?

The main goal for anyone with diabetes is to keep their blood glucose level within the normal range and minimize long-term health problems. To do this, the right food in the right amounts plus regular exercise and weight control is essential. If you are overweight, a weight loss of as little as 5 percent will help improve our blood glucose control, which will help reduce your risk of developing the complications of diabetes.

> **Dietary goals for people with diabetes**
> - less fat, especially the saturated kind
> - choose low glycemic index (GI) and wholegrain carbohydrate foods
> - choose lean meat, chicken, fish and their alternatives such as nuts and seeds
> - use low-fat dairy foods or their alternatives
> - eat only modest amounts of sugar and sugar-containing foods
> - use less salt
> - only drink alcohol in moderation if at all

Tips for eating a healthy, balanced diet when you have diabetes
What is healthy eating for diabetes?

Diabetes is a health problem that is greatly affected by the amount and types of food you eat. Therefore, a healthy diet is an essential part of its management. Advances in science mean there is now no such thing as a "diabetic" diet or one specific diet that suits everyone with diabetes. In fact, healthy eating guidelines recommended for the whole population also apply to people with diabetes.

Because everyone with diabetes is different, the finer points of these recommendations will vary from person to person. It is a good idea to take on the challenge of overhauling your diet with the guidance of a dietitian. A dietitian will ensure any advice is tailored to your individual needs and that, when possible, the foods you enjoy are still included in your diet plan.

Watch your fat intake, especially saturated fat

Too much fat won't help with weight control, and if you have diabetes the chances are you need to lose weight. Too much saturated and trans fat will also worsen insulin

What fat is that?

Fat	Where will you find it?
Saturated fats	butter, cream, palm oil, coconut milk and cream, fried foods and takeout, fat on meat and skin on chicken, full-fat dairy foods, deli meats and most commercial cakes, confectionery and cookies
Monounsaturated fat	olives and olive oil, avocados, peanuts and peanut oil, canola oil, macadamia nuts, hazelnuts, pecan nuts, cashew nuts and almonds
Omega-6 polyunsaturated fats	sunflower, safflower, soybean, sesame, cotton seed and grape seed oils, pine nuts and brazil nuts
Omega-3 polyunsaturated fats	oily types of fish—herring, sardine, mackerel, salmon and tuna; walnuts, canola oil, linseeds and linseed oil, lean red meat and a range of fortified commercial foods
Trans fats	margarines and fat spreads (some countries have less trans fats in these than others), deep-fried fast food, commercial cakes, pastries, pies and cookies

resistance, something you want to avoid if you want good blood glucose control. Therefore, of equal importance to the amount of fat you eat is the type of fat you eat. So, you need to control both the amount and types of fat you eat.

There are several different types of fats found in food. Some are healthy, some are not. Saturated fat makes insulin resistance worse and blood glucose harder to control. Saturated and trans fats increase your blood cholesterol level, which increases the risk of heart disease. When you have diabetes, your risk of heart problems is already higher than the average person. It is vital you use diet to help and not hinder in this regard.

It is important to make better choices about the types of fats you include in your diet. Small amounts of the healthier poly- and monounsaturated fats won't increase your blood cholesterol or worsen insulin resistance. This means that your blood vessels will stay in better shape and your blood glucose will be easier to control. Omega-3 fats also have unique health benefits when you have diabetes. They help keep your blood more fluid, reduce blood vessel inflammation and keep the heart beating more steadily. Eating oily fish at least three to four times a week will ensure you get enough of these valuable fats in your diet to reap their rewards.

Once you have made the switch to healthier fats, it is important to also consider ways of cutting down on your total fat intake. This is especially important if you are

15

Tips to reduce saturated fat
- avoid using butter, lard, cream, sour cream, coconut milk or cream and hard cooking margarines
- choose lean meat and trim fat before cooking
- always take the skin off chicken and other poultry
- eat cheese less often and choose lower fat varieties
- avoid high-fat processed deli meats like bologna and salami
- use low- or reduced-fat milk, yogurt, ice cream and custard
- avoid deep-fried takeout foods
- choose tomato-based sauces over creamy types
- eat less commercial cookies, cakes, pastries and sweets— save them for special occasions
- use low-fat cooking methods; steaming, grilling, baking and barbecuing

watching your weight or need to lose weight. See the tips on the left for the best ways to do this.

Healthy carbohydrates and the glycemic index

Carbohydrate foods are broken down into glucose after you eat them, providing your body with its main source of energy or fuel. Carbohydrates are the only part of the food you eat that will directly affect your blood glucose level, so the amount and type of carbohydrate you eat plays a big role in your blood glucose control.

Carbohydrates come in three forms: starch, sugar and fiber. These are found in varying proportions in different carbohydrate foods. Starches and sugars are digested to provide energy while fiber (which is largely undigested) keeps the digestive system healthy.

In the past, starches found in foods such as white bread, rice, potato and pasta were called "complex" carbohydrates because they are large and complex molecules. Sugars like glucose, sucrose, fructose and lactose were called "simple" carbohydrates because of their small and more simple structure.

Previously, scientists assumed that simple carbohydrates found in food would cause a greater rise in blood glucose than the complex carbohydrates. This was based on the assumption that the smaller sugars would be digested and absorbed faster than the larger starch molecules. This is the reason why people with diabetes were advised to avoid sugar. It was also assumed that the main factor in determining a carbohydrate's effect on blood glucose was the total amount you ate. Subsequently, people with diabetes were given long lists that showed different foods containing the same amount of carbohydrate that could be exchanged for one another in meals and snacks.

In the 1980s, when scientists actually measured blood glucose levels in people, they found that the amount of carbohydrate wasn't a good guide to a food's effect on blood glucose. Instead, it was the type of starch or sugar in the food that appeared to have the greatest influence. With this understanding came the realization that the terms "simple" and "complex" told us nothing about the way carbohydrates actually behave in the body.

Research into the effect of different carbohydrate foods on blood glucose has continued since these first studies in the 1980s. The Glycemic Index (GI) emerged from this research—a measure of the extent to which different carbohydrate foods and drinks

Typical blood glucose responses to high and low GI foods

This graph shows how the body's blood glucose response to high- and low-GI foods differs. Quickly-digested, high-GI foods produce a rush of glucose and insulin into the blood-stream followed by a large drop in blood glucose due to the action of insulin. In contrast, a low-GI food results in a smaller rise and fall in blood glucose.

cause the blood glucose level to rise after they have been eaten. The GI method assigns carbohydrate foods a number from 0 to 100 according to how they cause your blood sugar level to rise after eating them.

The GI method has shown that some carbohydrate foods like bread, rice and potatoes are digested and absorbed very quickly—far quicker than sugar—and as such have a much greater effect on your blood glucose level than was previously thought. High-GI foods are quickly digested and absorbed and produce a large, rapid rise in blood glucose. Low-GI foods are digested and absorbed more slowly resulting in a less dramatic and more steady blood glucose response and a lower insulin response. The effects of low-GI foods are what is preferred when you have diabetes.

It is difficult to predict the GI of a food just by looking at it, because there are several factors that affect the rate at which carbohydrate is digested:

- **Starch type:** some starches are digested more slowly than others. Foods that contain a greater proportion of slowly-digested starch will have a lower GI. For example, basmati rice and the newer, specially-bred doongara rice have a lower GI

GI ranking categories
Low-GI foods: less than 55
Medium-GI foods: 56 to 69
High-GI foods: greater than 70

than most other rice types because of its higher proportion of slower digested starch.

- **Starch particle size:** the processing of cereals from wholegrain to fine-milled grain makes starch particles smaller and easier to digest and increases their GI. This is why wholegrain breads have a lower GI than whole-wheat or finely-processed white bread and traditional wholegrain oats have a lower GI than quick-cooking oats.

- **Cooking:** this swells starch particles, making them more digestible and raising GI. Overcooked pasta will have a greater GI than when it is cooked *al dente*.

- **Fiber:** soluble fiber found in barley, oats, psyllium, legumes (lentils, chickpeas and dried beans) and some fruits slows digestion by increasing the thickness of food in the stomach.

- **Fat:** slows down food digestion and hence lowers GI. This should not be used as a green light to indulge in unhealthy high-fat foods like chocolate, potato chips, premium ice creams and croissants. Fatty foods, even if they're low GI, should be limited.

- **Protein:** makes it harder for digestive enzymes to reach starch particles and so slows their digestion. This partly explains why legumes have such a low GI.

- **Acid:** in certain amounts acid can slow food digestion. A salad with vinegar dressing can lower the GI of a meal because of this effect.

A low GI doesn't automatically make a food healthy (as in the case of high-fat foods) and a high-GI food is not always unhealthy. Many high-GI foods such as watermelon, cantaloupe and potatoes can still be eaten in moderation if you have diabetes. Simply enjoy them in smaller amounts, less frequently. Eating higher GI foods together with low-GI foods will also help lessen their impact on your blood glucose.

Eating low-GI foods as part of a healthy diet and lifestyle, when you have diabetes or prediabetes, has many health benefits to offer: lower blood cholesterol and triglycerides; a lower risk of heart problems; blood glucose can be better managed and your body's needs for insulin reduced; and weight loss is easier.

Achieving a lower GI diet is easy using the table of lower and higher GI foods on page 19. Start gradually by making one high-for-low GI food swap each day. Over time, increase the number of foods you swap to one at each meal or snack. You can also try "diluting" high-GI foods with low-GI foods; for example, have rice with lentils or kidney beans. You can also substitute lower GI ingredients in baking recipes, for example, using stoneground flour instead of refined white flour.

Good GI guide: The foods listed in this table are all healthy carbohydrate foods. However, by eating from the lower GI foods list more often you will find blood glucose control easier and weight more manageable.

HIGH VERSUS LOW GI

Type of food	Higher GI Versions	Lower GI Alternatives
Bread	Regular soft textured white, whole-wheat or rye bread and bread rolls, white or whole-wheat bagels, gluten-free bread, lebanese bread, melba toast, scones	Wholegrain breads with a relatively dense texture, pumpernickel bread, pita bread, sourdough bread, breads made from coarse, stoneground flour
Grains	Most types of rice (especially jasmine), millet, polenta (cornmeal)	Basmati rice, doongara rice, pearled barley, quinoa, buckwheat, bulgur (cracked wheat)
Pasta and noodles	Gluten-free corn or rice pasta, low-fat instant noodles, dried rice noodles, udon noodles, couscous	Durum wheat pasta—regular or protein-enriched, gluten-free legume-based pasta, mung bean noodles, fresh rice noodles, soba noodles, tortellini, ravioli
Breakfast cereals	Most processed breakfast cereals, including puffed grains (rice, amaranth, wheat, buckwheat), instant oatmeal, regular wheat breakfast biscuit cereals	Semolina, oatmeal made from whole or steel-cut oats, oat bran, natural muesli (without flakes), oat bran wheat biscuits
Biscuits and crackers *	Puffed crispbreads, water crackers, wafer crackers, plain sweet crackers, morning coffee biscuits	Cookies made with stoneground flour, whole rolled oats or whole grains with low-GI dried fruit
Vegetables and legumes **	Pumpkin, parsnips, tapioca; most potatoes—steamed, boiled, mashed (new potatoes have the lowest GI value out of the common varieties tested so far, but are still medium GI)	Sweet potato, yams, taro, green peas, carrots, sweet corn, all legumes (dried, boiled, canned, vacuum-packed); non-starchy vegetables (e.g. onions, tomatoes, lettuce, mushrooms, artichokes, asparagus, broccoli, cauliflower, ginger, garlic, cucumber, celery, pepper, leeks, herbs
Fruit	Cantaloupe, watermelon, sweetened dried cranberries, raisins, dried tenderized figs, lychees, canned in syrup, dark cherries, breadfruit, papaya	Apples, pears, stone fruit (raw or canned in natural juice), berries, bananas (the less ripe, the lower the GI), prunes, dried apples, apricots, peaches, pears, sultanas, kiwi fruit, mango, custard apple, citrus fruit, grapes
Dairy products and alternatives ***	Rice milk, sweetened condensed milk	Cows milk—plain or flavored, all types, soy milk—plain or flavored, all types, yogurt, ice cream, fromage frais

Some biscuits and crackers have low-GI values due to their high fat content and should not be eaten regularly.

** Most vegetables and herbs contain a little carbohydrate and don't produce a marked rise in blood glucose.

*** Dairy products that are sweetened with sugar have a higher GI value than those sweetened with a low-calorie sugar substitute.

19

Eat regular meals based on wholegrain and low-GI carbohydrate foods

Your diabetes will be easier to manage if you eat regular meals each day. For some this may mean three modest-sized meals—breakfast, lunch and dinner—while for others it may mean four to five smaller meals and snacks. Either way, it's best to avoid large amounts of carbohydrate-containing food at any one time of the day becaues this will make it harder for your body to keep your blood glucose level in the normal range.

Basing your meals on wholegrain, low-GI carbohydrate foods, lean protein, fruit, vegetables and healthy fats will help keep your blood glucose level in the normal range—and help keep hunger at bay.

For anyone with diabetes, especially if you need tablets or insulin, the advice of a dietitian is essential. A dietitian can help you work out the type of eating plan best suited to your health, medication and lifestyle needs.

Include lean protein foods

Protein foods are important for the maintenance and repair of body cells. These foods are also good sources of the minerals iron and zinc, and vitamins B12 and niacin. The best protein foods are lean meat, poultry, fish, eggs, nuts, legumes and seeds.

With all the hype over high-protein, low-carbohydrate diets and the belief that they promote weight loss, it is important to understand how these diets may harm your diabetes before you consider starting one. High-protein, low-carbohydrate diets should always be used with care when you have diabetes. This is especially so when you need insulin or tablets to manage your blood glucose.

Problems with high-protein, low-carbohydrate diets include:

• An increased risk of hypoglycemia (low blood glucose)

- An increased saturated fat intake which puts you at greater risk of high blood cholesterol levels and heart problems
- More protein in your diet may harm your kidneys, especially if they are already damaged.

However, if you are in good health and are finding your weight hard to shift, more lean protein and a little less carbohydrates on your plate may help, especially if the carbohydrate you eat is low GI. This isn't, however, a high-protein, low-carbohydrate diet. Consult with a dietitian for more advice if you are having trouble controlling your weight.

Low carbohydrate vegetables
Arugula
Asian greens e.g. bok choy, Chinese broccoli, choy sum
Asparagus
Bell peppers
Broccoli
Brussels sprouts
Cabbage
Cauliflower
Celery
Cucumber
Eggplant
Garlic
Leeks
Lettuce
Onions
Mushrooms
Radish
Spinach
Squash
Watercress
Zucchini

Watch the sugar and sugary foods
Too much sugar does not cause diabetes. People with diabetes no longer need to go to extreme lengths to avoid sugar like they used to. This is because research has shown us that sugar has a medium GI and has only a moderate effect on blood glucose (lower than some starchy foods like white or whole-wheat bread). Today, sugar is considered a part of a healthy diet for diabetes. However, it is still important to take care with added sugars as they are a source of extra calories.

A little brown sugar added to oatmeal, jam on grainy bread, or added sugar in low-fat yogurt are healthy ways to include sugar everyday and are unlikely to have a dramatic effect on your blood glucose level. (However, it is sensible to use "diet" varieties of foods like yogurt and jam sweetened with low-calorie sweeteners if you're trying to lose weight and are having difficulty keeping your blood glucose under control.) On the other hand, too much added sugar from non-diet soft drinks, fruit juice, chocolates, cakes and cookies probably will. These higher sugar foods are also more likely to contribute excess calories and make managing your weight much more difficult.

While it is not always necessary to use an alternative to sugar, there is still a place for sweeteners and sweetened foods in your diet when you have diabetes. However,

using diet products and low-calorie sweeteners more often than sugar-sweetened versions is still a good idea. Baking is also a good opportunity to use sweeteners, such as sucralose, and there are several products available that replace sugar spoon for spoon to give equal sweetness but with less calories.

Eat more vegetables and legumes

Everyone needs at least five servings of vegetables every day. Unfortunately, most of us don't eat enough, and if you have diabetes you are probably no exception. Increasing your vegetable intake has several benefits:

- It will help you feel full with fewer calories—if you need to cut back on your food intake and have a big appetite, try a leafy salad with a low-fat dressing as an entrée.
- You will eat more fiber, which helps improve regularity and blood glucose and cholesterol levels
- It will help protect your eyes and blood vessels from the damage caused by high blood glucose levels—the antioxidants and other protective phytochemicals in vegetables, herbs, spices and fruits have been shown to help protect our eyes.

Don't hold back, load up your plate at every opportunity. Low-carbohydrate types are best, especially if you need to manage your weight, and, the brighter the color the better for important protective antioxidants and phytochemicals.

Shop smart

Being a smart shopper and choosing the healthiest foods for you requires some skill in reading food labels.

Fat: Choose foods that are lowest in fat and don't forget to check out their saturated fat levels. Occasionally it is okay to choose higher fat foods if their saturated fat is very low and they mostly contain poly- or monounsaturated fats.

Sugar: The total amount of sugar in a food includes added sugars and those occurring naturally such as that from fruit or milk. Go for lower sugar foods where you can.
Fiber: Always choose foods with the most fiber. High fiber foods have 3 g of fiber per serving while very high fiber foods have 6 g or more fiber per serving.
Salt: Look for salt-reduced or no-added-salt foods wherever you can. As a guide foods with less

than 120 mgs of sodium per 100 g are good choices.
GI: Choose foods with oats, wholegrains, nuts, seeds, rice bran or oat bran, dried fruit. Also, keep an eye out for the GI symbol on foods but consider their fat and calorie content before you buy. Not all processed, low-GI foods are helpful for weight control.

Legumes such as lentils, chickpeas, soybeans and kidney beans are nutritious, low-GI and high in fiber and antioxidants and should be a staple in your pantry—and can easliy be added to soups, casseroles and salads.

Keep salt down

Too much salt can raise your blood pressure, increasing your risk of heart and kidney problems. Simply avoiding adding salt while cooking or to your meals is not enough. Around 75 percent of the salt in our diets comes from processed foods.

To keep salt down, look for reduced-salt or no-added-salt versions of the foods you normally buy. You will most commonly find lower salt alternatives for margarine spreads, canned tomatoes, tomato paste, tomato sauce, baked beans, crackers, peanut butter, cheese and cooking stocks or sauces. Always drain and rinse tinned legumes and buy fish in water, not brine or oil.

Avoiding obviously salty foods, such as bacon, ham, olives, canned fish in brine, salted nuts and chips will also help keep your salt intake down.

Enjoy alcohol in moderation

Alcohol guidelines for people with diabetes are similar to those for people without diabetes: two standard drinks a day for men and one for women. However, if you have diabetes, it is always better to enjoy alcohol with a meal or some carbohydrate food.

Alcohol is high in calories making it harder to manage your weight. It also increases triglycerides (a type of blood fat) and blood pressure and can cause your blood glucose to go dangerously low (a hypo) if you use insulin or tablets to control your diabetes. Therefore, it is better for your health and blood glucose control if you watch your alcohol intake and reduce it where you can.

Before considering the place of alcohol in your life, discuss its pros and cons with your doctor, diabetes educator or dietitian. This is especially important if you use tablets or insulin to manage your diabetes, as alcohol may not be safe unless you are combining it with the right amounts of carbohydrates.

Simple tips to cut back on alcohol include:

- Reducing your thirst before you drink alcohol with water or diet drinks
- Drink low-alcohol beer
- Alternate alcoholic and non-alcoholic drinks
- Dilute alcoholic drinks with soda or water

Exercise, a final word . . .

A cookbook is obviously about what you eat. However, no advice about health, diet and weight is complete without some mention of physical activity. If you have or are at risk of diabetes then becoming more physically active is vital to achieving the lifestyle you need to optimize your health.

Advantages to being more physically active include:

- Better insulin sensitivity so your body needs less insulin
- Lowers blood pressure
- Helps lower blood cholesterol
- Makes weight control easier
- Reduces stress
- Strengthens your bones and muscles
- Makes you feel good

For advice on the amount and type of physical activity you need it is best to consult

with your doctor, exercise physiologist or diabetes educator. These health professionals are most able to consider what exercise is appropriate for you given your medical background and current level of fitness.

Being aware of how active you are in your normal daily routine can also help you make changes to how you do things. Investing in a pedometer will tell you about the number of steps you take each day. The more steps you take, the more physically active you become. Think of ways to increase your daily physical activity, such as:

- Taking the stairs rather than the elevator or escalator
- Parking a little further away from the doors at the shopping mall
- Walking to get the paper rather than taking the car
- Getting up to turn the TV off rather than using the remote
- Making a regular date with a friend to go for a walk.

How to use this book

The recipes in this book have all been selected because of the valuable contribution they make to healthy eating. Any higher fat recipes are rich in heart-friendly monounsaturated or polyunsaturated fats. Where possible the recipes are also high in fiber and contain low glycemic index (GI) carbohydrates to make blood glucose levels easier to manage. All of the recipes are low in saturated fat to help reduce your risk of heart desease.

Disclaimer

The information in this book is intended to provide people with diabetes, and people who care for them, with general advice about healthy low-GI eating (accurate at the time of printing). This advice may not be sufficient for some people with multiple health problems or serious complications. It is not intended to replace any advice given to you by a qualified doctor or other mainstream health professional. It is important that diabetes is diagosed by a doctor, using standard diagnostic tests (blood samples, biopsies and assessment of your symptoms). Neither the author nor the publishers can be held responsible for claims arising from the inappropriate use or incorrect interpretation of any of the dietary advice described in this book.

Note: Many recipes call for self-rising flour. If you cannot find this in your supermarket, you can use all-purpose flour and add 1½ teaspoons baking powder for each cup of flour used.

BREAKFAST

HOMEMADE MUESLI

NATURAL MUESLI PROVIDES A HEALTHY MIX OF NUTRIENTS AND DELICIOUS FLAVORS. SERVED WITH FRESH FRUIT, MILK OR YOGURT IT'S A GREAT WAY TO START THE DAY.

2 cups old fashioned rolled oats

2 tbsp wheat germ

¼ cup unprocessed wheat
  bran or oat bran

½ cup dried apricots,
  chopped

½ cup dried apple, chopped

⅓ cup golden raisins

½ cup slivered raw almonds

low-fat milk, to serve

PREP TIME: 10 MINUTES
COOKING TIME: NONE
SERVINGS: 8

Combine the rolled oats, wheat germ, wheat bran, dried fruit and almonds in a bowl and mix well. Store in an airtight container until ready to use.

Serve the muesli with low-fat milk.

HINTS:
- This muesli can be stored in an airtight container for up to 4 weeks.
- It will be low GI as long as you use rolled oats, not quick-cooking oats. You can substitute the almonds with Brazil nuts, hazelnuts or pecans.
- To save preparation time, you can buy a packet of chopped dried fruit medley to use instead of the apricot, apple and sultanas. Replace the sultanas with lower GI dried pear, peach or prunes, if you prefer.
- For some low-GI serving suggestions, try low-fat yogurt or fresh low-GI fruit, such as berries, apple, pear, peach, plum, apricot or nectarine.

nutrition per serving: Energy 201 Cal; Fat 6.2 g; Saturated fat 0.7 g; Protein 5.5 g; Carbohydrate 28.2 g; Fiber 5.4 g; Cholesterol 0 mg

BIRCHER MUESLI

IF YOUR REGULAR MUESLI IS A BIT HO-HUM, TRY THIS ONE. IT'S NOT ONLY DELICIOUS, IT'S LOW GI, FILLING AND A GOOD SOURCE OF SOLUBLE FIBER AND PRODUCES A RANGE OF VITAMINS AND MINERALS.

3 cups old-fashioned rolled oats
1 cup low-fat milk
⅓ cup low-fat plain yogurt
½ cup freshly squeezed, unsweetened orange juice
about 2 cups mixed seasonal fresh low-GI fruit, such as ripe banana, peach, pear, plum, apple or berries
2 apples, grated
½ cup low-fat plain yogurt, extra

1 tbsp pure maple syrup, to serve (optional)

PREP TIME: 15 MINUTES + 4 HOURS REFRIGERATION
COOKING TIME: NONE
SERVINGS: 6

Combine the oats, milk, yogurt and orange juice in a bowl and mix well. Cover and refrigerate for 4 hours, or overnight.

Serve with the low-GI fresh fruit of your choice, grated apple and extra yogurt. Drizzle with a little maple syrup, if desired.

HINTS:
• Make sure you use wholegrain oats, not quick-cooking ones.
• You can also add ½ cup slivered almonds. This will increase the fat and energy content, but the fat will be mostly the unsaturated type.
• For extra flavor you can add the grated apple to the oat mix and then store it in the fridge overnight.

nutrition per serving: Energy 298 Cal; Fat 4.5 g; Saturated fat 0.8 g; Protein 10 g; Carbohydrate 51.3 g; Fiber 5.6 g; Cholesterol 3 mg

OATMEAL

1 cup old fashioned rolled oats
½ cup low-fat milk, plus extra to serve

PREP TIME: 5 MINUTES
COOKING TIME: 10 MINUTES
SERVINGS: 2

Mix the oats with 1½ cups of cold water in a small heavy-based saucepan. Stir in the milk and bring to a boil. Cook for about 7 minutes, stirring constantly, until thick and creamy. Serve immediately.

Serve the oatmeal with low-fat milk. It is delicious with a dried fruit compote (see recipe on page 35).

HINTS:
- The coarser the oats, the lower the GI. When choosing oats, avoid instant or quick-cooking oats—these are not low GI. Choose the traditional wholegrain, slow-cooking oats instead. If you can't find wholegrain oats in the supermarket, look for them in your local health food shop. You could also use steel cut oats or Scotch oats.
- For a delicious fruity oatmeal, stir 2 tablespoons of chopped dried apricots into the mixture for the last 3 minutes of cooking. Some other low-GI serving suggestions to try are stewed apple, grated pear or apple, wheat germ, oat bran (a good source of soluble fiber), dried apricots, dried apples, prunes or low-fat yogurt.
- If you need to add some sweetener, use some low-GI fruit or a little yellow box honey, pure maple syrup or low-calorie sweetener.

OATMEAL IS A SUSTAINING BREAKFAST AND ESPECIALLY NICE TO WARM YOU UP ON COLD WINTER MORNINGS. USE TRADITIONAL SLOW-COOKING OATS INSTEAD OF INSTANT OR QUICK-COOKING OATS TO KEEP THIS MEAL LOW GI.

nutrition per serving: Energy 219 Cal
Fat 4.3 g
Saturated fat 0.8 g
Protein 8.1 g
Carbohydrate 34.5 g
Fiber 3.4 g
Cholesterol 3 mg

33

FRESH FRUIT SALAD

THIS LOW-GI FRESH FRUIT SALAD CAN BE ENJOYED AS A LIGHT MEAL ON ITS OWN—TOPPED WITH SOME LOW-FAT PLAIN YOGURT AND SUNFLOWER SEEDS OR GROUND FLAX SEEDS—OR IT CAN BE ADDED TO MUESLI OR EATEN AS A SNACK.

2 pears, cored and cut into cubes
2 apples, cored and cut into cubes
¾ cup strawberries, hulled and halved
¾ cup blueberries
2 oranges, peeled, seeded and cut into cubes
2 kiwi fruit, peeled and cut into cubes
¼ cup seedless white grapes

2 just-ripe bananas, sliced
3 tbsp unsweetened fruit juice or freshly squeezed orange juice

PREP TIME: 1O MINUTES
COOKING TIME: NONE
SERVINGS: 4

Prepare the fruit just prior to serving. Combine the chopped fruits in a bowl, pour over the fruit juice or orange juice and toss to coat.

HINT:
• You can substitute any seasonal low-GI fruits, such as peaches or mandarins.

nutrition per serving: Energy 218 Cal; Fat 0.4 g; Saturated fat 0 g; Protein 3.4 g; Carbohydrate 46.6 g; Fiber 8.6 g; Cholesterol 0 mg

DRIED FRUIT COMPOTE WITH YOGURT

THIS FRUITY BREAKFAST IS FULL OF FLAVOR AND IS A GREAT SOURCE OF FIBER, CALCIUM AND POTASSIUM. IT ALSO PROVIDES SOME ANTIOXIDANTS, SUCH AS BETACAROTENE. DON'T OVERDO IT THOUGH, IT'S NOT LOW IN CALORIES!

⅓ **cup dried apricots, quartered**
¼ **cup pitted prunes, quartered**
⅓ **cup dried pears, chopped**
⅓ **cup dried peaches, chopped**
¾ **cup freshly squeezed orange juice**
1 cinnamon stick
low-fat plain yogurt, to serve

PREP TIME: 5 MINUTES
COOKING TIME: 10 MINUTES
SERVES 4

Put the fruit, orange juice and cinnamon stick in a saucepan over medium heat and stir to combine. Bring to a boil, then reduce the heat to low. Cover and simmer for 10 minutes, or until the fruit is plump and softened. Discard the cinnamon stick. Serve drizzled with the cooking liquid and a dollop of the plain yogurt.

Store in an airtight container in the refrigerator for up to 1 week.

HINT:
• This is a healthy recipe, but people with diabetes should not have large servings because it is an energy-dense food.

nutrition per serving: Energy 125 Cal; Fat 0.2 g; Saturated fat 0 g; Protein 1.9 g; Carbohydrate 27.1 g; Fiber 4.1 g; Cholesterol 0 mg

THIS DISH IS A FANTASTIC ALTERNATIVE
TO BREAKFAST CEREAL OR OATMEAL
AND IS A GOOD WAY TO ADD QUINOA
(PRONOUNCED KEEN-WA) TO YOUR
DIET.

nutrition per serving: Energy 362 Cal

Fat 3.4 g

Saturated fat 0.3 g

Protein 11.9 g

Carbohydrate 64.6 g

Fiber 9 g

Cholesterol 2 mg

MIXED BERRY QUINOA

1 cup quinoa, rinsed and drained

2 cups unsweetened apple and
    blackcurrant juice

1 cinnamon stick

2 cups raspberries

1²/₃ cups blueberries

1²/₃ cups strawberries, hulled and halved

2 tsp lime or lemon zest, plus extra

1 tbsp finely shredded mint

³/₄ cup low-fat plain or fruit-flavored yogurt
    (see Hint)

1 tbsp pure maple syrup (optional)

PREP TIME: 10 MINUTES + REFRIGERATION
    TIME

COOKING TIME: 15 MINUTES

SERVINGS: 4–6

Put the apple and blackcurrant juice and quinoa into a saucepan and add the cinnamon stick. Bring to a boil, then cover and simmer for 12–15 minutes, or until quinoa is translucent and the juice has been absorbed. Remove the cinnamon stick. Transfer to a large bowl, cover and refrigerate until cold.

Add the berries, lime or lemon zest and mint to the quinoa and gently fold through. Spoon the mixture into 4 bowls. Top with a large dollop of yogurt and a little maple syrup, if desired. Serve chilled.

HINT:
• Flavored yogurt with no added sugar has less carbohydrate and calories in it and a lower GI than sugar-sweetened yogurt.

POACHED EGGS WITH SPINACH

THIS EASY RECIPE GIVES YOU A NEW TWIST ON POACHED EGGS WITH MORE FLAVOR AND NUTRIENTS, AND FAR LESS FAT THAN EGGS BENEDICT. IT'S AN IDEAL MEAL TO ENJOY WITH FRIENDS ON LAZY WEEKENDS.

DRESSING
½ **cup low-fat plain yogurt**
1 small garlic clove, crushed
1 tbsp chopped chives

about 10 oz baby spinach leaves
1 scant tablespoon reduced-fat olive or
   canola oil margarine

4 tomatoes, halved
1 tbsp white vinegar
8 eggs
8 thick slices wholegrain bread, toasted

PREP TIME: 10 MINUTES

COOKING TIME: 15 MINUTES

SERVES 4

To make the dressing, mix together the yogurt, garlic and chives.

Wash the spinach and put it in a large saucepan with just the little water that is left clinging to the leaves. Cover the pan and cook over low heat for 3–4 minutes, or until the spinach has wilted. Add the margarine, then season with freshly ground black pepper and toss together. Remove the pan from the heat and keep warm.

Put the tomatoes, cut side up, under a preheated grill (broiler) and grill for 3–5 minutes, or until softened and warm.

Fill a deep frying pan three-quarters full with cold water and add the vinegar to stop the egg whites spreading. Bring the water to a gentle simmer. Gently break an egg into a small bowl, then carefully slide into the water, then repeat with the remaining eggs. Reduce the heat so that the water barely moves. Cook for 1–2 minutes, or until the eggs are just set. Remove with a spatula. Drain on paper towels.

Top each slice of toast with some spinach, an egg and some dressing. Serve with the tomato halves. Season with pepper if desired.

nutrition per serving: Energy 439 Cal; Fat 16.1 g; Saturated fat 4 g; Protein 26.1 g; Carbohydrate 42.3 g; Fiber 8.3 g; Cholesterol 377 mg

MUSHROOMS WITH SCRAMBLED EGGS AND TOMATOES

THIS IS A CLASSIC BREAKFAST AND FILLING AS WELL! IT PROVIDES GOOD AMOUNTS OF PROTEIN, VITAMIN A, IRON AND FOLATE.

4 field mushrooms
olive or canola spray oil
4 roma (plum) tomatoes, halved
3 tbsp balsamic vinegar
4 eggs, lightly beaten
4 egg whites, lightly beaten
3 tbsp low-fat milk

2 tbsp snipped chives
8 thick slices wholegrain bread

PREP TIME: 10 MINUTES
COOKING TIME: 15 MINUTES
SERVINGS: 4

Trim the mushroom stalks to ¾ in above the cap. Wipe the mushrooms with paper towels to remove any dirt and grit.

Spray both sides of the mushrooms with the oil and place on a non-stick baking tray with the tomatoes. Drizzle the mushrooms and tomatoes with the balsamic vinegar, then sprinkle with freshly ground black pepper and place under a medium grill (broiler) for 10–15 minutes, or until tender.

Meanwhile, put the eggs, egg whites, milk and chives in a bowl and whisk together to combine. Pour the mixture into a non-stick frying pan and cook over low heat for 2–3 minutes, or until the egg begins to set, then gently stir with a wooden spoon to scramble.

Toast the wholegrain bread until golden brown, then cut on the diagonal. Serve with the mushrooms, tomato and scrambled egg.

HINTS:
- Use omega-3 enriched eggs instead of regular eggs to improve the fat profile of this dish. Omega-3 enriched eggs are available in most large supermarkets and some health food shops.
- People with diabetes are at high risk of developing heart disease (much higher than people without diabetes). So it's important that they don't add salt to their meals.

nutrition per serving: Energy 334 Cal; Fat 8.5 g; Saturated fat 2 g; Protein 20.8 g; Carbohydrate 39.5 g; Fiber 6.1 g; Cholesterol 188 mg

RICOTTA CORN FRITTERS

7 oz low-fat ricotta cheese

1 egg

1 egg white

½ cup skim milk

½ cup whole-wheat, self-rising flour

15 oz canned corn kernels, drained

3 spring onions (scallions), chopped

2 tbsp snipped chives

olive or canola oil spray

3½ oz low-fat ricotta cheese, extra

⅓ cup salsa

PREP TIME: 10 MINUTES

COOKING TIME: 25 MINUTES

MAKES 4

Combine the ricotta, egg, egg white and milk in a bowl and beat until smooth. Stir in the flour, corn kernels, spring onion and chives. Season well with freshly ground black pepper.

Spray a non-stick frying pan with the oil. Add heaped tablespoons of the mixture to the pan, four at a time, and flatten to about ⅝ in thick. Cook for 3–4 minutes each side. Drain on paper towels.

Serve the fritters in a stack of three and top with a tablespoon of ricotta cheese and a tablespoon of salsa.

HINTS:
• Use stoneground, whole-wheat flour to help reduce the GI of this dish.
• You could also serve with some grilled tomatoes, mushrooms, spinach and wholegrain bread for a more filling meal.

A NICE CHOICE FOR A SAVORY
BREAKFAST—THIS DELICIOUS,
REDUCED-FAT FRITTER RECIPE IS A
GREAT SOURCE OF PROTEIN, CALCIUM,
VITAMIN A AND B VITAMINS.

nutrition per serving: Energy 297 Cal
Fat 7.2 g
Saturated fat 2.2 g
Protein 15.6 g
Carbohydrate 39.7 g
Fiber 5.4 g
Cholesterol 48 mg

HERB OMELETTE

THIS NOURISHING OMELETTE IS READY IN A FLASH AND IS DELICIOUS AT ANY TIME OF THE DAY. THE COMBINATION OF PROTEIN AND LOW-GI CARBOHYDRATE MAKES IT VERY SUSTAINING.

4 eggs

2 tbsp finely chopped flat-leaf (Italian) parsley

2 tbsp chopped chives

olive or canola oil spray

⅓ cup low-fat, grated cheddar cheese

4 thick slices wholegrain bread, toasted

fresh cherry tomatoes, to serve

PREP TIME: 10 MINUTES

COOKING TIME: 5 MINUTES

SERVINGS: 2

Break the eggs into a large bowl and whisk with a fork. Whisk in 2 tablespoons of water, then add the parsley and chives. Season with freshly ground black pepper.

Spray a small non-stick frying pan with the oil. Heat over hgh heat, then reduce the heat to medium and add half of the omelette mixture. Swirl with a fork several times.

While the mixture is cooking, tilt the pan and lift the edge of the omelette occasionally to allow the uncooked egg to flow underneath. When the mixture is half cooked, sprinkle with half of the grated cheese, then leave to cook a little more (the base should be golden brown and the inside nearly set). Using a spatula, fold the omelette in half in the pan. Flip it over onto a warm plate.

Gently re-whisk the remaining egg mixture, then cook in the same way as this first. Serve with the toast and fresh cherry tomatoes.

nutrition per serving: Energy 408 Cal; Fat 15.6 g; Saturated fat 4.6 g; Protein 27.7 g; Carbohydrate 37 g; Fiber 4.5 g; Cholesterol 382 mg

HOMEMADE BAKED BEANS

HEALTHIER THAN TINNED BAKED BEANS, THIS DISH IS A DELICIOUS WAY TO INCLUDE MORE LEGUMES IN YOUR DIET. BEANS ARE RICH IN FIBER AND POTASSIUM AND THE TOMATOES ARE A GOOD SOURCE OF ANTIOXIDANTS.

3 cups dried kidney beans
1²/₃ cups no-added salt tinned diced tomatoes
1 cup reduced-salt vegetable or chicken stock
1 bay leaf
2 tbsp chopped flat-leaf (Italian) parsley

pinch of dried thyme
1 tbsp olive or canola oil

PREP TIME: 5 MINUTES + 8 HOURS SOAKING
COOKING TIME: 2 HOURS 10 MINUTES
SERVES 4

Wash the beans and place in a large bowl. Cover with 6 cups water and soak for 8 hours, or overnight. Drain.

Cook the kidney beans in a saucepan filled with plenty of water for about 1½ hours, or until tender. Drain. Preheat the oven to 350°F.

Put the beans in a casserole dish and add the tomato, stock, herbs and oil. Bake, covered, for 40 minutes.

Serve the baked beans with grainy toast or grainy muffins spread with a little low-fat cottage cheese topped with fresh spinach and season with pepper.

HINT:
• If you want a thicker consistency, remove the lid of the casserole dish and cook for a further 10–15 minutes, or until reduced to the desired consistency. Instead of using dried kidney beans, you can use the same amount of drained, canned kidney beans.

nutrition per serving: Energy 462 Cal; Fat 8 g; Saturated fat 1.1 g; Protein 31.2 g; Carbohydrate 57.9 g; Fiber 27.7 g; Cholesterol 1 mg

THIS NOURISHING MEAL IS A GOOD
SOURCE OF MANY NUTRIENTS
INCLUDING PROTEIN, B-GROUP
VITAMINS AND ANTIOXIDANTS. SERVE
WITH WHOLEGRAIN BREAD FOR A
BALANCED LOW-GI MEAL.

nutrition per serving: Energy 350 Cal
Fat 15.6 g
Saturated fat 3.9 g
Protein 15 g
Carbohydrate 36.5 g
Fiber 5.4 g
Cholesterol 187 mg

EGGS EN COCOTTE

TOMATO SAUCE

1 tbsp olive or canola oil

1 garlic clove, crushed

3 vine-ripened tomatoes (about 10½ oz),
   peeled, seeded and chopped

½ tsp olive or canola oil

4 eggs

Tabasco sauce, to taste

2 tbsp snipped fresh chives

8 slices thick wholegrain bread

1 tbsp reduced-fat olive or canola oil
   margarine

PREP TIME: 15 MINUTES

COOKING TIME: 30 MINUTES

SERVINGS: 4

Preheat the oven to 180°F. To make the tomato sauce, heat the oil in a heavy-based frying pan. Add the garlic and cook for 1 minute, or until it begins to turn golden. Add the tomato and season with some freshly ground black pepper. Cook over medium heat for 15 minutes, or until thickened.

Grease four ½ cup ramekins with the oil, then break 1 egg into each, trying not to break the yolk. Pour the sauce around the outside of each egg so the yolk is still visible. Add a little tabasco sauce, sprinkle with the chives and season with pepper, if desired.

Place the ramekins in a deep baking dish and pour in enough hot water to come halfway up the side of the ramekins. Bake for 7–10 minutes, or until the egg white is set. Toast the bread and lightly spread with the margarine. Serve immediately with the egg.

SCRAMBLED TOFU WITH MUSHROOMS

THIS IS A NOURISHING LOW-GI BREAKFAST THAT PROVIDES GOOD AMOUNTS OF PROTEIN, FIBER, FOLATE AND IRON.

1 tbsp reduced-fat olive or canola oil margarine
7 oz button mushrooms, sliced
1 garlic clove, crushed
2 spring onions (scallions), chopped
14 oz firm tofu, drained and crumbled
1 tsp reduced-sodium soy sauce

1 tbsp finely chopped, flat-leaf (Italian) parsley
8 thick slices soy and linseed bread

PREP TIME: 10 MINUTES
COOKING TIME: 15 MINUTES
SERVES 4

Melt half of the margarine in a large frying pan. Add the mushrooms and cook over high heat for 5 minutes, or until they start to lose their moisture. Add the garlic and cook for 5 minutes, or until the liquid has evaporated. Remove from the pan.

Melt the remaining margarine in the pan. Add the spring onion and cook for 30 seconds, or until just wilted. Add the tofu, soy sauce and mushrooms and cook, stirring gently, for 2 minutes, or until the tofu is heated through. Stir in the parsley and season with freshly ground black pepper.

Lightly toast the bread and serve with the scrambled tofu.

HINT:
• Add some tomatoes and spinach if you want some more flavor and color.

nutrition per serving: Energy 364 Cal; Fat 16.7 g; Saturated fat 2.6 g; Protein 26.4 g; Carbohydrate 26.4 g; Fiber 7.8 g; Cholesterol 0 mg

SUMMER ORANGE JUICE

THIS REFRESHING BLEND OF CITRUS AND STONE-FRUIT JUICES IS A RICH SOURCE OF FOLATE, POTASSIUM AND THE ANTIOXIDANTS BETACAROTENE AND VITAMIN C.

3 oranges, peeled
5 small plums, pits removed
4 peaches, pits removed
10 apricots, pits removed

PREP TIME: 10 MINUTES
COOKING TIME: NONE
SERVES 2

Juice the oranges, plums, peaches and apricots in a juice extractor or blender. Stir well to combine.

HINT:
• Enjoy this juice in moderation if you are watching your weight. Fresh fruit is more filling than fruit juice. The general recommendation for adults and kids is to drink no more than one juice drink a day.

nutrition per serving: Energy 360 Cal; Fat 1.2 g; Saturated fat 0 g; Protein 7.5 g; Carbohydrate 67.4 g; Fiber 15 g; Cholesterol 0 mg

BANANA SMOOTHIE

2 just-ripe bananas
¼ cup low-fat vanonela or fruit-flavored
   yogurt
2 cups low-fat milk
2 tbsp wheat germ or oat bran
freshly grated nutmeg, to taste

PREP TIME: 5 MINUTES
COOKING TIME: NONE
SERVES 2

Put the bananas in a blender or food processor. Add the yogurt, milk, wheat germ and nutmeg. Blend or process until smooth, then pour into two chilled glasses.

HINTS:
- The GI of bananas increases as the fruit ripens, so choose bananas that have only just ripened.
- You can substitute the bananas with other low-GI fruit, such as berries, pears, apricots, plums, peaches or nectarines.
- Choose a flavored yogurt with no added sugar. Check the ingredients list and look for one that has been sweetened with a low-calorie sweetener, such as aspartame, rather than sugar.
- Choose calcium-enriched, low-fat milk for a calcium boost.

THIS LOW-GI, CALCIUM-RICH SMOOTHIE IS GOOD FOR YOUR TEETH AND BONES AND MAKES A DELICIOUS LIGHT BREAKFAST.

nutrition per serving: Energy 219 Cal
Fat 1 g
Saturated fat 0.5 g
Protein 14.3 g
Carbohydrate 37.1 g
Fiber 3.4 g
Cholesterol 10 mg

BREAKFAST SMOOTHIE

THIS REFRESHING SMOOTHIE PROVIDES SOME CARBOHYDRATE AND PROTEIN TO HELP ENERGIZE YOUR BRAIN AND BODY AND IMPROVE YOUR MOOD. IT'S VERY EASY TO MAKE AND EVEN EASIER TO DRINK.

5½ oz fresh low-GI fruit, such as peach,
   plum, pear, or strawberries
¼ cup low-fat vanilla yogurt
1 cup low-fat milk
1 tbsp malted milk powder
2 tsp wheat germ or oat bran
1 egg (optional)

PREP TIME: 5 MINUTES
COOKING TIME: NONE
SERVES 2

Put the fruit in a blender or food processor. Add the yogurt, milk, milk powder, wheat germ and egg (if you are using it). Blend or process until well combined, then pour into two chilled glasses.

HINTS:
- Experiment with various low-GI fruits to work out your favorite combination for this low-fat smoothie.
- There are many types of yogurt on the market. Choose a low-fat diet yogurt that contains a low-calorie sweetener instead of sugar. Diet yogurt that is sweetened with aspartame or a similar low-calorie sweetener has a lower GI and less calories than yogurt sweetened with sugar.

nutrition per serving: Energy 143 Cal; Fat 3.3 g; Saturated fat 1.1 g; Protein 11.4 g; Carbohydrate 16.3 g; Fiber 1.4 g; Cholesterol 101 mg

CARROT, APRICOT AND NECTARINE JUICE

ONE VEGETABLE AND TWO FRUITS COMBINE TO MAKE THIS DELICIOUS AND NUTRITIOUS DRINK, RICH IN ANTIOXIDANTS.

2 lb 4 oz baby carrots
10 apricots, pits removed
4 large nectarines, pits removed
ice cubes, to serve
lemon slices, to serve

PREP TIME: 10 MINUTES
COOKING TIME: NONE
SERVES 2

Juice the carrots, apricots and nectarines in a juice extractor or use a blender. Stir to combine and serve over ice with lemon slices.

nutrition per serving: Energy 450 Cal; Fat 1.5 g; Saturated fat 0 g; Protein 10.9 g; Carbohydrate 81 g; Fiber 25 g; Cholesterol 0 mg

SNACKS AND LIGHT MEALS

THIS LOW-CALORIE DIP IS DELICIOUS AS
A SNACK WITH CRUNCHY RAW VEGETABLE
STICKS OR AS A LOW-FAT SUBSTITUTE
FOR MAYONNAISE OR MARGARINE IN
SANDWICHES AND BURGERS.

nutrition per serving: Energy 22 Cal
Fat 0.1 g
Saturated fat 0.04 g
Protein 2.2 g
Carbohydrate 2.5 g
Fiber 0.4 g
Cholesterol 2 mg

TZATZIKI

2 cucumbers

1²/₃ cups low-fat plain yogurt

4 garlic cloves, crushed

**3 tbsp finely chopped mint, plus extra,
   to garnish**

1 tbsp lemon juice

PREP TIME: 10 MINUTES +
   15 MINUTES STANDING

COOKING TIME: NONE

SERVES 12

Cut the cucumbers in half lengthways, scoop out the seeds and discard. Leave the skin on and coarsely grate the cucumber into a small colander. Sprinkle with salt and leave over a large bowl for 15 minutes to drain off any bitter juices.

Meanwhile, combine the yogurt, garlic, mint and lemon juice.

Rinse the cucumber under cold water then, taking small handfuls, squeeze out any excess moisture. Combine the grated cucumber with the yogurt mixture and season well with freshly ground black pepper. Garnish with mint. Serve with vegetable sticks.

HINTS:
• Tzatziki will keep in an airtight container in the fridge for 2–3 days.
• To make vegetable sticks, cut raw carrots, celery, zucchini and unpeeled cucumbers into 2³/₄ in sticks, and raw cauliflower and broccoli into small florets.

CANNELLINI BEAN AND CHICKPEA DIP

THIS LOW-GI DIP IS A DELICIOUS AND EASY WAY TO EAT BEANS AND CHICKPEAS. ENJOY AS A SNACK WITH FRESH VEGETABLES OR AS A SPREAD ON BREAD.

15 oz canned cannellini (white) beans, rinsed and drained
15 oz canned chickpeas, rinsed and drained
1½ tsp ground cumin
3 garlic cloves, crushed
2 tbsp chopped flat-leaf (Italian) parsley
3 tbsp lemon juice
1 tsp lemon zest
1 tbsp tahini

PREP TIME: 10 MINUTES
COOKING TIME: NONE
SERVES 3–4

Put all the ingredients in a food processor and process for 30 seconds. With the motor still running, slowly add 3 tablespoons hot water to the processor in a thin stream until the mixture is smooth and "dippable." Serve at room temperature with vegetable sticks and pita crisps.

HINT:
• Tahini is a thick paste made of ground sesame seeds. It is available at large supermarkets and health food shops.

nutrition per serving (4): Energy 175 Cal; Fat 4.9 g; Saturated fat 0.7 g; Protein 10.8 g; Carbohydrate 18.7 g; Fiber 8.8 g; Cholesterol 0 mg

HUMMUS

THIS POPULAR DIP IS A GREAT SOURCE OF FIBER, FOLATE AND POTASSIUM AS WELL AS BEING DELICIOUS.

1 cup dried chickpeas
3 tbsp olive oil
3–4 tbsp lemon juice
2 garlic cloves, crushed
2 tbsp tahini
1 tbsp ground cumin

PREP TIME: 15 MINUTES + 8 HOURS SOAKING
COOKING TIME: 1 HOUR
SERVES 2–4

Soak the chickpeas in water for 8 hours, or overnight. Drain. Put in a saucepan, cover with cold water, bring to a boil and cook for about 50–60 minutes. Drain, reserving ¾–1 cup of the cooking liquid.

Place the chickpeas in a food processor with the oil, lemon juice, garlic, tahini and cumin. Blend well until the mixture begins to look thick and creamy. With the motor running, gradually add the reserved cooking liquid until the mixture reaches the desired consistency. Serve with toasted wholegrain bread, pita bread, vegetable sticks or use as a spread on sandwiches.

nutrition per serving: Energy 398 Cal; Fat 23.4 g; Saturated fat 3 g; Protein 13.1 g; Carbohydrate 25 g; Fiber 11.3 g; Cholesterol 0 mg

RICE PAPER ROLLS WITH SHRIMP

20 large, cooked shrimp, peeled and
  deveined
1 small carrot
1 cucumber
1¾ cups finely shredded red cabbage
 8 spring onions (scallions)
1 handful mint, torn
2 handfuls cilantro leaves
8 x 6 in square rice paper wrappers

DRESSING
½ cup lime juice
2 tbsp sweet chili sauce
3 garlic cloves, crushed
1 long red chili, seeded, finely chopped
2 tsp grated palm sugar or

  brown sugar
1 tbsp rice vinegar
1 tbsp fish sauce
2 tbsp chopped cilantro leaves and stems

PREP TIME: 20 MINUTES

COOKING TIME: NONE

MAKES 20 (SERVES 4–6)

Cut the shrimp into ½ in slices, on the diagonal. Julienne the carrot into 1½ in lengths. Cut the cucumber into ½ in lengths. Thinly slice the spring onions diagonally. Put the shrimp, cabbage, carrot, cucumber, spring onions, mint and coriander in a large bowl and toss to combine.

To make the dressing, combine all the dressing ingredients in a small bowl and mix well. Pour ⅓ cup of the dressing over the prawn mixture and toss to combine. Working with one wrapper at a time, dip into a bowl of hot water for 10 seconds, or until softened, drain, then lay out on a flat surface.

Place ¼ cup of the mixture on one side of the wrapper, leaving a border at the sides. Fold in the sides and roll up tightly. Cover with a damp cloth and repeat with the remaining filling and wrappers to make 20 rolls. Serve with the remaining dressing as a dipping sauce.

HINT:
• Although delicious, these rice paper rolls should be enjoyed in moderation as the rice paper itself is medium GI. They are, however, low in fat.

THESE ROLLS ARE A GREAT SOURCE OF
FOLATE AND THE ANTIOXIDANTS
BETACAROTENE AND VITAMIN C. THE
SHRIMP PROVIDE IODINE AND
SELENIUM—MINERALS MOST PEOPLE
DON'T EAT ENOUGH OF.

nutrition per serving (4): Energy 317 Cal
Fat 1.5 g
Saturated fat 0.3 g
Protein 24.5 g
Carbohydrate 47.9 g
Fiber 3.9 g
Cholesterol 150 mg

59

STUFFED PEPPERS

MEDITERRANEAN-STYLE FLAVORS ENHANCE THE RICE, HAM AND VEGETABLE FILLING IN THE BAKED PEPPERS. THIS COLORFUL MEAL IS LOW GI AND RICH IN ANTIOXIDANTS AND POTASSIUM.

1 eggplant, peeled and diced
1 onion, finely chopped
2 garlic cloves, chopped
15 oz canned no-added-salt diced
   tomatoes
1 tsp sugar
1 tbsp dried thyme
1 tsp dried oregano
2 cups cooked brown basmati rice
1¾ oz chopped, low-fat ham (we used 97%
   fat-free) (optional)
4 oz canned corn kernels, drained
olive or canola oil spray

4 red peppers, halved and seeded
½ cup grated, low-fat cheddar cheese

PREP TIME: 25 MINUTES
COOKING TIME: 1 HOUR 5 MINUTES
SERVES 4

Preheat the oven to 350°F. Place the eggplant, onion, garlic and ½ cup of water in a large, deep, heavy-based frying pan. Bring to a boil, then lower the heat, cover and simmer for 8 minutes, or until softened. Stir once or twice. Remove the lid and simmer until any remaining liquid has evaporated.

Add the tomatoes, sugar and herbs and season well with pepper. Simmer, uncovered, for 8 minutes. Remove from the heat and stir in the rice, ham and corn.

Spray the pepper shells on the outside with the oil. Fill the pepper halves with the mixture. Put the peppers in a large baking dish, pour 1 cup of water into the dish, cover with foil and bake for 45 minutes, or until the peppers have softened. Remove the foil and sprinkle each pepper half with grated cheese. Bake for a further 5 minutes, or until the cheese has melted. Serve with a mixed green salad dressed with vinegar.

HINT:
• You need ¾ cup uncooked brown rice to make 2 cups cooked brown rice.

nutrition per serving: Energy 296 Cal; Fat 4.5 g; Saturated fat 1.3 g; Protein 14.6 g; Carbohydrate 45.6 g; Fiber 6.6 g; Cholesterol 11 mg

CORN AND PEPPER FRITTERS

JUST LIKE SPANISH OMELETTE, THESE FRITTERS CAN ALSO BE SERVED COLD FOR A PICNIC OR PARTY. TRY SERVING THEM WITH A LOW-FAT DIPPING SAUCE.

1 large red pepper

2–3 cobs fresh corn kernels or 1½ cups canned corn kernels, drained

olive or canola oil, for frying

2 tbsp chopped flat-leaf (Italian) parsley, cilantro leaves, chives or dill

3 eggs

PREP TIME: 20 MINUTES

COOKING TIME: 10 MINUTES

SERVES 4

Cut the pepper into large pieces, discarding the seeds and membrane, then chop into small pieces. Cut the kernels from the fresh corn, using a sharp knife. Heat 2 tablespoons of oil in a frying pan. Add the corn and stir over medium heat for 2 minutes. Add the pepper and stir for a further 2 minutes. Transfer the vegetables to a bowl. Add the herbs and stir well to combine. Beat the eggs in a small bowl with a little freshly ground black pepper. Stir the egg gradually into the vegetable mixture.

Heat a non-stick frying pan over medium heat. Add enough oil to cover the base. Drop large spoonfuls of the vegetable mixture into the oil, a few at a time. Cook the fritters for 1–2 minutes, or until brown. Turn and cook the other side. Drain on paper towels and keep warm while you cook the remainder.

HINTS:
- These fritters may be served with some wholegrain bread and a green salad for lunch, or as an accompaniment to a main course.
- Take care as these fritters contain no flour, so they cook quickly. You want them to still be a little creamy in the middle when done.

nutrition per serving: Energy 238 Cal; Fat 6.8 g; Saturated fat 1.5 g; Protein 11.3 g; Carbohydrate 29.4 g; Fiber 6.8 g; Cholesterol 141 mg

THESE PIZZAS ARE A MUCH BETTER
CHOICE THAN COMMERCIAL ONES AND A
GOOD EXAMPLE OF HOW YOU CAN STILL
ENJOY YOUR FAVORITE FOODS IN
MODERATION IF YOU HAVE DIABETES.

nutrition per serving: Energy 431 Cal
Fat 9.4 g
Saturated fat 4.7 g
Protein 25 g
Carbohydrate 58.8 g
Fiber 8.5 g
Cholesterol 28 mg

PITA PIZZAS

4 large whole-wheat pita pockets
½ cup 99% fat-free tomato salsa
½ red onion, thinly sliced
3¼ oz mushrooms, thinly sliced
2¼ oz low-fat ham (we used 97% fat-free),
　thinly sliced
½ cup black olives in brine, rinsed, drained,
　pitted and chopped
1 tbsp capers, rinsed, drained and chopped
½ cup low-fat feta cheese

¼ cup sprigs rosemary
1 cup grated light (reduced-fat) mozzarella

PREP TIME: 15 MINUTES
COOKING TIME: 20 MINUTES
SERVES 4

Preheat the oven to 400°F. Place the pita breads on a large baking tray or on two smaller trays. Spread each with the salsa. Scatter over the onion, mushrooms, ham, olives and capers.

Crumble over the feta and top with the rosemary sprigs and mozzarella. Bake for 20 minutes. Serve immediately.

VARIATIONS:
• Use no-added-salt tomato pasta sauce or salsa sauce on the base, then choose from the following toppings: low-fat ham, pineapple pieces, sliced pepper, onion or olives marinated in brine.
• For a meaty topping, try leftover savory minced (ground) beef or spaghetti bolognaise and low-fat cheddar cheese.
• For a little spice, try salami, corn kernels, sliced green pepper, onion, tomato and low-fat feta cheese.
• A tasty vegetarian option is artichoke hearts, tomato and zucchini slices, ricotta and low-fat feta cheese.
• An easy seafood version uses tuna in springwater, sliced mushroom and pepper, and low-fat cheddar cheese.

HINT:
• Look for pita pockets made from stoneground flour as they are lower GI.

CORN AND BACON CRUSTLESS QUICHES

FOR AN OCCASIONAL TREAT, THESE REDUCED-FAT QUICHES ARE DELICIOUS—ALL THE FLAVOR BUT
LESS FAT THAN REGULAR QUICHES.

4 corn cobs
1 tsp olive or canola oil
**4 slices low-fat bacon slices (we used 97%
   fat-free), cut into thin strips**
1 small onion, finely chopped
3 eggs, lightly beaten
2 tbsp chopped chives
2 tbsp chopped flat-leaf (Italian) parsley
¾ cup fresh wholegrain breadcrumbs
4 tbsp skim evaporated milk

PREP TIME: 30 MINUTES
COOKING TIME: 40 MINUTES
MAKES 4

Preheat the oven to 350°F. Lightly grease four ¾ cup ramekins. Remove the husks from
the corn and, using a coarse grater, grate the corn kernels into a deep bowl. There should
be about 1½ cups corn flesh and juice.

Heat the oil in a frying pan and cook the bacon and onion for 3–4 minutes, or until the
onion softens. Add to the corn in the bowl. Stir in the eggs, chives, parsley, breadcrumbs
and evaporated milk and season well with freshly ground black pepper. Spoon into the
ramekins.

Put the ramekins in a large baking dish. Add enough hot water to come halfway up the sides
of the ramekins. Lay foil loosely over the top. Bake for 25–30 minutes, or until just set.

nutrition per serving: Energy 282 Cal; Fat 7.4 g; Saturated fat 1.9 g; Protein 17.2 g; Carbohydrate 35.1 g;
Fiber 4.9 g; Cholesterol 149 mg

ITALIAN OMELETTE

IF YOU FIND PLAIN OMELETTES A BIT BORING, THIS ITALIAN-FLAVORED VERSION IS THE THING FOR YOU. SERVE WITH WHOLEGRAIN BREAD FOR A COMPLETE, MORE FILLING LOW-GI MEAL.

5½ oz fusilli
1 tsp olive or canola oil
1 onion, finely chopped
4½ oz low-fat ham, sliced
6 eggs
3 tbsp low-fat milk
¼ cup grated parmesan cheese
2 tbsp chopped flat-leaf (Italian) parsley
1 tbsp chopped basil
olive or canola oil spray

½ cup grated, low-fat cheddar cheese
wholegrain bread, to serve

PREP TIME: 20 MINUTES
COOKING TIME: 25 MINUTES
SERVES 4

Cook the pasta in a large saucepan of boiling water for 10 minutes, or until *al dente*. Drain and cool.

Heat the oil in a non-stick frying pan. Add the onion and stir over low heat for 5 minutes, or until tender. Add the ham and stir for 1 minute. Transfer to a plate.

Whisk together the eggs and milk and season well with freshly ground black pepper. Stir in the pasta, parmesan, herbs and onion mixture.

Preheat the grill or broiler. Heat the frying pan and spray with oil. Pour the egg mixture into the pan. Sprinkle with the cheddar. Cook over medium heat until the omelette begins to set around the edges, then put the pan under the grill until the omelette is set and lightly browned on top. Cut into wedges and serve with wholegrain bread.

HINTS:
• You can use any short durum wheat pasta.
• Durum wheat pasta has a low-GI value. However, it should not be overcooked. Overcooking pasta until it is soft and soggy makes its starch more digestible and increases its GI value. Pasta should be served *al dente*.

nutrition per serving: Energy 350 Cal; Fat 13.7 g; Saturated fat 4.9 g; Protein 27.7 g; Carbohydrate 28 g; Fiber 1.7 g; Cholesterol 308 mg

MUSHROOM AND SPINACH FRITTATA

olive or canola oil spray

1 red onion, thinly sliced

1¾ oz low-fat bacon (we used 97% fat-
free), thinly sliced

3 garlic cloves, crushed

3¼ oz mushrooms, thinly sliced

2 zucchini, diced

1 handful baby spinach leaves

4 eggs

¼ cup skim or non-fat milk

½ cup grated low-fat cheddar cheese

2 tbsp shredded parmesan cheese

2 tbsp basil, thinly shredded

PREP TIME: 20 MINUTES

COOKING TIME: 25 MINUTES + COOLING TIME

SERVES 4

Spray a large non-stick frying pan with oil. Heat the oil, add the onion, bacon and garlic and stir-fry for 4 minutes, or until soft. Add the mushrooms and zucchini and stir-fry for 3 minutes, or until the mushrooms are cooked and any liquid has evaporated. Stir in the spinach and cook until just wilted. Cool.

Whisk together the eggs and milk in a large bowl. Stir in the cheeses, basil and cooled vegetable mixture.

Take a non-stick frying pan with a diameter of 7–8 in (across the base) and spray with oil. Pour in the mixture and smooth the surface. Cook over low heat for 10–13 minutes, or until mostly set. Take care not to burn the base.

Preheat a grill or broiler to medium. Place the pan under the grill and cook for 3–5 minutes, or until firm and lightly browned on top. Serve warm or cold, cut into slices. Season with pepper and serve with a balsamic-dressed salad.

FRITTATAS ARE A FILLING LIGHT MEAL AND TASTY TO BOOT! THIS ONE'S A GOOD SOURCE OF CALCIUM, PROTEIN AND VITAMINS A, B AND D.

nutrition per serving: Energy 171 Cal
Fat 9.1 g
Saturated fat 3.3 g
Protein 18 g
Carbohydrate 3.9 g
Fiber 2.3 g
Cholesterol 200 mg

CHICKPEA FRITTERS

THESE LOW-GI FRITTERS ARE AN EXCELLENT SOURCE OF FIBER AND PROVIDE A GOOD AMOUNT OF PROTEIN TOO.

2 tsp olive or canola oil
4 spring onions (scallions), sliced
2 garlic cloves, finely chopped
1 small red chili, seeded and finely
  chopped
21 oz canned chickpeas, rinsed and drained
2 tbsp chopped cilantro
1 egg, lightly beaten
olive or canola oil spray
99% fat-free tomato salsa, to serve

3½ oz mixed salad leaves, to serve
wholegrain bread, to serve

PREP TIME: 20 MINUTES
COOKING TIME: 25 MINUTES
MAKES 6

Preheat the oven to 400°F. Line a baking tray with baking paper. Heat 2 teaspoons of the oil in a large non-stick frying pan over medium heat. Add the spring onions, garlic and chili and cook, stirring, for 1–2 minutes, or until the spring onion softens.

Put the chickpeas and spring onion mixture and coriander in a food processor. Process until the mixture just starts to hold together. Do not overprocess—the mixture should be just roughly processed. Transfer to a bowl and mix in the egg. Using wet hands, shape the mixture into six even fritters.

Lightly spray the fritters with spray oil and put on prepared tray. Bake for 20 minutes turning once until lightly golden brown. Serve with salsa, mixed lettuce and bread.

nutrition per fritter (6): Energy 103 Cal; Fat 4.3 g; Saturated fat 0.7 g; Protein 5.5 g; Carbohydrate 9.1 g; Fiber 3.6 g; Cholesterol 31 mg

BAKED SWEET POTATOES MEXICANA

LIKE SOME SPICE? THIS DISH IS THE PERFECT HOT POTATO! IT CONTAINS CARBOHYDRATES, FIBER AND ANTIOXIDANTS. TOP WITH LOW-FAT SOUR CREAM OR YOGURT FOR EXTRA CALCIUM.

4 medium sweet potatoes
olive or canola oil spray
1 garlic clove, crushed
1 onion, finely chopped
9 oz lean ground beef
**10½ oz canned red kidney beans, rinsed
  and drained**
1 tbsp no-added-salt tomato paste

½ cup 99% fat-free, mild tomato salsa
**extra light sour cream or low-fat yogurt, to
  serve**

PREP TIME: 20 MINUTES
COOKING TIME: 40 MINUTES
SERVES 4

Preheat the oven to 400°F. Prick the sweet potatoes a few times with a skewer. Bake on the oven rack for 40 minutes, or until cooked through.

Meanwhile, heat a non-stick frying pan over medium heat. Lightly spray with the oil. Add the garlic and onion and cook for 2–3 minutes, or until softened. Add the beef and cook, breaking up any lumps with a wooden spoon, for 5 minutes, or until browned. Drain off any excess fat. Stir in the kidney beans, tomato paste and salsa. Bring to a boil, then reduce the heat and simmer for 10 minutes, or until slightly thickened.

Make a deep cut along the top of each cooked sweet potato. Divide the mixture among them and top with a dollop of extra-light sour cream or low-fat yogurt, if you like.

nutrition per serving: Energy 322 Cal; Fat 5.8 g; Saturated fat 2 g; Protein 21.1 g; Carbohydrate 41.8 g; Fiber 8.5 g; Cholesterol 32 mg

SOUPS AND SALADS

THIS CLASSIC SOUP IS LOW GI AND
LOW-FAT. IT IS ALSO A GOOD SOURCE OF
POTASSIUM, BETACAROTENE AND
LYCOPENE.

nutrition per serving: Energy 126 Cal
Fat 3 g
Saturated fat 0.5 g
Protein 7.6 g
Carbohydrate 15.1 g
Fiber 4.1 g
Cholesterol 6 mg

TOMATO SOUP

2 tsp olive or canola oil
1 celery stalk, finely chopped
1 onion, finely chopped
1 carrot, finely chopped
2 garlic cloves, crushed
28 oz canned chopped tomatoes
3 cups reduced-salt chicken or vegetable
   stock
1 tbsp no-added-salt tomato paste
1 parsley sprig

1 bay leaf
1 cup low-fat milk
3 tbsp finely chopped flat-leaf (Italian)
   parsley
wholegrain toast, to serve

PREP TIME: 15 MINUTES
COOKING TIME: 25 MINUTES
SERVINGS: 4

Melt the oil in a saucepan and sauté the celery, onion and carrot for 3–4 minutes. Add the garlic and cook for 30 seconds. Add the chopped tomatoes, chicken or vegetable stock, tomato paste, parsley sprig and bay leaf. Bring to a boil, then simmer for 15 minutes. Remove the parsley and bay leaf.

Purée the soup coarsely in a blender, then return it to the pan. Stir through the milk and heat until hot.

Garnish with the parsley and serve with toasted wholegrain bread.

ROASTED RED PEPPER SOUP

ROASTED RED PEPPERS AND TOMATOES ARE A GREAT FLAVOR COMBINATION AND MAKE THIS
VEGETARIAN SOUP A RICH SOURCE OF THE ANTIOXIDANT BETACAROTENE.

4 large red peppers
4 ripe tomatoes
2 tsp olive or canola oil
1 red onion, chopped
1 garlic clove, crushed
4 cups reduced-salt vegetable stock
1 tsp sweet chili sauce
parmesan cheese, to serve

flat-leaf (Italian) parsley, to serve
6 thick slices wholegrain bread

PREP TIME: 30 MINUTES
COOKING TIME: 45 MINUTES
SERVINGS: 6

Cut the peppers into large flat pieces, removing the seeds and membrane. Put skin side up under the broiler until blackened. Leave covered with a dish towel until cool, then peel away the skin and chop the flesh.

To peel the tomatoes, score a cross in the base of each one. Cover with boiling water for 30 seconds, then plunge into cold water. Drain and peel away the tomato skin from the cross. Cut in half, scoop out the seeds and roughly chop the flesh.

Heat the oil in a large frying pan and add the onion. Cook over medium heat for 10 minutes, stirring frequently, until very soft. Add the garlic and cook for a further minute. Add the pepper, tomato and stock. Bring to a boil, reduce the heat and simmer for about 20 minutes.

Coarsely purée the soup in a food processor or blender (in batches if necessary). Return to the pan to reheat gently and stir in the chili sauce. Top with fresh parsley and shavings of parmesan cheese. Serve with sliced wholegrain bread.

nutrition per serving: Energy 174 Cal; Fat 3.5 g; Saturated fat 0.5 g; Protein 6.7 g; Carbohydrate 26.6 g; Fiber 5 g; Cholesterol 0 mg

SPLIT PEA SOUP

A GREAT WAY TO INCLUDE LEGUMES IN YOUR DIET, THIS DELICIOUS LOW-GI SOUP PROVIDES SOLUBLE FIBER, FOLATE, B-GROUP VITAMINS AND MINERALS.

2 tbsp olive or canola oil
1 large brown onion, chopped
1 large carrot, cut into ½ in cubes
1 large celery stick, cut into ½ in cubes
2 bay leaves
1 tbsp thyme, finely chopped
6 garlic cloves, finely chopped
2 cups yellow split peas

4 cups reduced-salt chicken stock
¼ cup lemon juice

PREP TIME: 20 MINUTES
COOKING TIME: 1 HOUR 20 MINUTES
SERVINGS: 6–8

Heat the oil in a large saucepan over medium heat. Add the onion, carrot and celery, and cook for 4–5 minutes, or until starting to brown. Add the bay leaves, thyme and garlic and cook for 1 minute.

Stir in the split peas, then add the chicken stock and 4 cups water. Cook for 1 hour 15 minutes, or until the split peas and vegetables are soft. Stir often during cooking to prevent the soup from sticking to the bottom of the pan, and skim any scum from the surface. Add a little extra water if the soup is too thick.

Remove the soup from the heat and discard the bay leaves. Stir in the lemon juice and season with freshly ground black pepper.

nutrition per serving (8): Energy 236 Cal; Fat 5.9 g; Saturated fat 0.8 g; Protein 14.6 g; Carbohydrate 28.4 g; Fiber 6.5 g; Cholesterol 1 mg

MEDITERRANEAN FISH SOUP

½ tsp saffron threads

2 tsp olive or canola oil

2 large onions, thinly sliced

1 leek, chopped

4 garlic cloves, finely chopped

1 bay leaf, torn

½ tsp dried marjoram

1 tsp grated orange zest

2 tbsp dry white wine (optional)

1 red pepper, cut into bite-sized pieces

about 1 lb ripe tomatoes, chopped

½ cup puréed tomatoes (see Hints)

2 cups reduced-salt fish or vegetable stock

2 tbsp no-added-salt concentrated purée

1 tsp brown sugar

about 1 lb skinless and boneless fish fillets, trimmed and cut into bite-sized pieces (see Hints)

3 tbsp chopped flat-leaf (Italian) parsley

4 wholegrain bread rolls or slices

PREP TIME: 30 MINUTES

COOKING TIME: 45 MINUTES

SERVINGS: 4

Soak the saffron threads in a small bowl with 2 tablespoons of boiling water.

Heat the oil in a large saucepan over low heat. Add the onion, leek, garlic, bay leaf and marjoram. Cover and cook for 10 minutes, shaking the pan occasionally until the onion is soft. Add the zest, wine, pepper and tomato, cover and cook for 10 minutes.

Add the puréed tomatoes, stock, tomato paste, sugar and saffron (with the liquid) to the pan. Stir well and bring to a boil, then reduce the heat to low and simmer, uncovered, for 15 minutes.

Add the fish to the soup, cover and cook for 8 minutes, or until tender. Add half the parsley, then season with freshly ground black pepper. Discard the bay leaf. Sprinkle the soup with the remaining parsley just before serving.

Warm the bread, then serve with the soup.

HINTS:
- Italian tomato purée is available in jars at supermarkets.
- Try snapper, red mullet, red rock cod or ocean perch.

THIS SOUP EVOKES THE WARMTH OF THE
MEDITERRANEAN AND IS A GREAT WAY TO INCLUDE
FISH IN YOUR DIET. IT'S A GOOD SOURCE OF
PROTEIN, ANTIOXIDANTS, B-GROUP VITAMINS AND
MINERALS, AND IS LOW IN FAT.

nutrition per serving: Energy 381 Cal
Fat 6.4 g
Saturated fat 1.1 g
Protein 34.4 g
Carbohydrate 40.2 g
Fiber 8.4 g
Cholesterol 54 mg

COUNTRY-STYLE VEGETABLE SOUP

A SATISFYING LOW-GI MEAL THE WHOLE FAMILY WILL ENJOY, THIS SOUP IS ALSO AN EASY WAY TO INCLUDE LEGUMES AND A VARIETY OF DIFFERENT VEGETABLES IN YOUR DIET.

1 cup soup mix or pearl barley
2 tsp olive or canola oil
1 leek, thinly sliced
2 garlic cloves, finely chopped
1 green pepper, chopped
2 zucchini, sliced
2 celery stalks, sliced
4½ oz button mushrooms, sliced
2 carrots, sliced
2 orange sweet potatoes, peeled and chopped

8 cups reduced-salt vegetable stock
1 bunch broccoli, cut into small florets
1 large handful flat-leaf (Italian) parsley, finely chopped

PREP TIME: 25 MINUTES + OVERNIGHT SOAKING
COOKING TIME: 1 HOUR
SERVINGS: 6

Put the soup mix or barley in a large bowl, cover with water and leave to soak for 8 hours, or overnight. Drain and rinse well.

Heat the oil in a large saucepan and cook the leek and garlic for 5 minutes, or until soft. Add the pepper, zucchini, celery and mushrooms and cook for 5 minutes, or until starting to become soft. Add the carrot, sweet potato and barley and stir well.

Pour in the stock and bring to a boil. Reduce the heat to low, partially cover the pan with a lid and simmer for 45 minutes, or until the vegetables and barley are just soft. Add the broccoli florets and cook a further 5 minutes until broccoli is just cooked. Sprinkle with parsley and season with freshly ground black pepper to serve. For a thinner soup add a little water.

HINTS:
• The soup will keep for 2 days in the refrigerator or in the freezer for 1 month. Bring to a boil before serving.

nutrition per serving: Energy 231 Cal; Fat 3.7 g; Saturated fat 0.7 g; Protein 8.1 g; Carbohydrate 36.7 g; Fiber 11.9 g; Cholesterol 27 mg

BEAN AND SAUSAGE SOUP

SOUP IS A GREAT WAY TO WARM UP ON A COLD WINTER'S NIGHT. THIS ONE IS RICH AND HEARTY AND WILL SATISFY THE WHOLE FAMILY.

¼ cup olive or canola oil

4 low-fat beef sausages

2 leeks, sliced

1 garlic clove, crushed

1 large carrot, chopped into small cubes

2 celery stalks, sliced

2 tbsp all-purpose flour

8 cups reduced-salt beef stock

½ cup white wine (see Hints)

1½ cups small pasta shells

14 oz canned three-bean mix, drained and rinsed (see Hints)

1 tsp chopped fresh chili (optional)

PREP TIME: 25 MINUTES

COOKING TIME: 30 MINUTES

SERVINGS: 4–6

Heat the oil in a large heavy-based saucepan and add the sausages. Cook over medium heat for 5 minutes, or until golden, turning regularly. Drain the cooked sausages on paper towels, and then dice.

Add the leek, garlic, carrot and celery to the pan and cook, stirring occasionally, for 2–3 minutes, or until soft.

Add the flour and cook, stirring, for 1 minute. Add the stock and wine and bring to a boil, then reduce the heat and simmer for 10 minutes.

Add the pasta, beans and chili (if using) to the pan. Increase the heat and cook for 8–10 minutes, or until the pasta is *al dente*. Return the sausage to the soup and season to taste with freshly ground black pepper. Serve with some low-GI wholegrain bread and a mixed salad for a complete meal.

HINTS:
- If you'd prefer not to use wine, the same amount of liquid can be replaced with reduced-salt beef stock.
- You can use dried beans, if you prefer. Put them in a large bowl, cover with water and leave to soak overnight. Drain and rinse well, then transfer to a large saucepan with enough water to come about 1¼ in above the beans. Bring to a simmer and cook for 1 hour. Drain well before adding to the soup. Boiled dried beans have a slightly lower GI value than canned beans.They also have a denser texture, making them slightly more filling.

nutrition per serving (6): Energy 230 Cal; Fat 5.3 g; Saturated fat 1.5 g; Protein 11.7 g; Carbohydrate 27.8 g; Fiber 6.1 g; Cholesterol 4 mg

THIS IS A GREAT RECIPE FOR BUSY
PEOPLE—IT CAN BE PREPARED IN LESS
THAN 30 MINUTES IF YOU HAVE ALL THE
INGREDIENTS ON HAND, GIVING YOU A
QUICK, FILLING, LOW-GI MEAL.

nutrition per serving: Energy 332 Cal
Fat 3.1 g
Saturated fat 0.9 g
Protein 33 g
Carbohydrate 40 g
Fiber 3.8 g
Cholesterol 88 mg

THAI-STYLE CHICKEN AND CORN SOUP

4 cups reduced-salt chicken stock

15 oz canned corn kernels, undrained

8 spring onions (scallions), sliced

1 tbsp finely chopped fresh ginger

about 1 lb lean, skinless chicken breast,
   trimmed and thinly sliced

1 tbsp sweet chili sauce

1 tbsp fish sauce

7 oz fresh thin rice noodles

2 large handfuls cilantro leaves, chopped

2 tsp grated lime zest

2 tbsp lime juice

PREP TIME: 15 MINUTES

COOKING TIME: 10 MINUTES

SERVINGS: 4

Bring the stock to a boil in a large saucepan over high heat. Add the corn kernels and their juice, spring onion and ginger, then reduce the heat and simmer for 1 minute.

Add the chicken, sweet chili sauce and fish sauce and simmer for 3 minutes, or until the chicken is cooked through.

Put the noodles in a large heatproof bowl, cover with boiling water and soak for 5 minutes, or until softened. Separate gently and drain.

Add the noodles, cilantro, lime zest and lime juice to the soup and serve immediately.

MINESTRONE PRIMAVERA

THIS SOUP CELEBRATES THE RETURN OF SPRING WITH A MIX OF FRESH GREEN VEGETABLES. IT IS
A GOOD SOURCE OF FIBER, FOLATE, POTASSIUM AND BETACAROTENE.

1 tbsp olive or canola oil
4 to 5 low-fat bacon slices (we used 97% fat-free), finely chopped
2 onions, chopped
2 garlic cloves, thinly sliced
2 small celery stalks, sliced
8 cups reduced-salt chicken stock
⅓ cup macaroni
2 zucchini, chopped
2 cups shredded savoy cabbage
1 cup frozen peas
1 cup green beans, trimmed and chopped
1 cup shredded spinach leaves

14 oz canned cannellini beans, drained and rinsed
1 large handful basil, chopped
grated parmesan cheese, to serve

PREP TIME: 25 MINUTES
COOKING TIME: 40 MINUTES
SERVINGS: 4–6

Heat the oil in a large saucepan. Add the bacon, onion, garlic and celery and cook over low heat for 8 minutes, stirring occasionally until the vegetables are soft but not brown. Add the stock and bring to a boil. Simmer, covered, for 10 minutes.

Add the macaroni and boil for 12 minutes, or until almost *al dente*. Stir in the zucchini, cabbage, peas and beans and simmer for 5 minutes. Add the spinach, cannellini beans and basil and simmer for 2 minutes. Season with freshly ground black pepper and serve with the grated parmesan.

nutrition per serving (6): Energy 196 Cal; Fat 4.3 g; Saturated fat 0.8 g; Protein 14.9 g; Carbohydrate 21.9 g; Fiber 7.6 g; Cholesterol 10 mg

ASPARAGUS AND MUSHROOM SALAD

THIS STYLISH SALAD IS IDEAL AS A STARTER OR AS A SIDE DISH WITH MEAT OR FISH. THE
FLAVORS AND TEXTURES OF THE MUSHROOMS AND ASPARAGUS COMPLEMENT EACH OTHER
PERFECTLY.

6 oz asparagus, trimmed
1 tbsp wholegrain mustard
1 tbsp grated orange zest
2 tsp grated lemon zest
2 tsp grated lime zest
3 tbsp orange juice
2 tbsp lemon juice
1 tbsp lime juice
2 garlic cloves, crushed
1 tsp sugar

14 oz button mushrooms, halved
5½ oz arugula
1 red pepper, cut into strips

PREP TIME: 20 MINUTES
COOKING TIME: 10 MINUTES
SERVINGS: 4

Snap the woody ends from the asparagus spears and cut in half on the diagonal. Cook in boiling water for 1 minute, or until just tender. Drain, plunge into cold water and set aside.

Put the mustard, citrus zest and juice, garlic and sugar in a large saucepan and season with freshly ground black pepper. Bring to a boil, then reduce the heat and add the mushrooms, tossing for 2 minutes. Cool.

Remove the mushrooms from the sauce with a slotted spoon. Return the sauce to the heat, bring to a boil, then reduce the heat and simmer for 3–5 minutes, or until reduced. Cool slightly.

Toss the mushrooms, arugula, pepper and asparagus together. Put on a plate and drizzle with the sauce.

nutrition per serving: Energy 73 Cal; Fat 0.8 g; Saturated fat 0.01 g; Protein 6.4 g; Carbohydrate 7.1 g; Fiber 4.5 g; Cholesterol 0 mg

WARM SHRIMP, ARUGULA AND FETA SALAD

about 2 lbs raw shrimp

4 spring onions (scallions), chopped

4 roma (plum) tomatoes, chopped

1 red pepper, chopped

14 oz canned chickpeas, drained and rinsed

1 tbsp chopped dill

3 tbsp finely shredded basil

1 tbsp extra virgin olive oil

1 tbsp reduced-fat olive or canola oil
   margarine

2 small fresh red chilies, finely chopped

4 garlic cloves, crushed

2 tbsp lemon juice

10½ oz arugula

4½ oz low-fat feta cheese

PREP TIME: 30 MINUTES

COOKING TIME: 10 MINUTES

SERVINGS: 4–6

Peel the shrimp, leaving the tails intact. Gently pull out the dark vein from each shrimp back, starting at the head end.

Combine the spring onion, tomato, pepper, chickpeas and herbs in a bowl and mix well.

Heat the oil and margarine in a large frying pan or wok. Add the shrimp and cook, stirring, over high heat for 3 minutes. Add the chili and garlic, and continue cooking until the shrimp turn pink. Remove from the heat and stir in the lemon juice.

Arrange the arugula leaves on a large platter, top with the tomato mixture, then the shrimp mixture. Crumble the feta cheese over the top.

HINT:
• If serving as a main meal enjoy this salad with some wholegrain bread or stoneground, whole-wheat pita bread, a bean salad or basmati rice.

THIS COLORFUL LOW-GI SALAD WILL
IMPRESS YOUR FRIENDS AND FAMILY
AND IS SUITABLE AS A STARTER OR A
MAIN MEAL.

nutrition per serving (6): Energy 246 Cal
Fat 10.5 g
Saturated fat 3 g
Protein 26.7 g
Carbohydrate 9.1 g
Fiber 4 g
Cholesterol 128 mg

SPICY LENTIL SALAD

LENTILS, LIKE ALL LEGUMES, ARE A NATURAL SUPER FOOD—THEY'RE LOW GI, A GREAT SOURCE OF FIBER, AND PROVIDE GOOD AMOUNTS OF VITAMINS, MINERALS AND ANTIOXIDANTS.

1 cup heaping basmati rice
1 cup brown lentils
1 tsp ground turmeric
1 tsp ground cinnamon
6 cardamom pods
3 star anise
2 bay leaves
3 tbsp olive or canola oil
1 tbsp lemon juice
1 cup broccoli florets
2 carrots, peeled and cut into julienne strips
1 onion, finely chopped
2 garlic cloves, crushed
1 red pepper, finely chopped

1 tsp garam masala
1 tsp ground coriander
1²⁄₃ cups fresh or frozen peas, thawed if frozen

DRESSING
1 cup low-fat plain yogurt
1 tbsp lemon juice
1 tbsp chopped mint
1 tsp cumin seeds

PREP TIME: 30 MINUTES
COOKING TIME: 1 HOUR 15 MINUTES
SERVINGS: 6

Put the rice, lentils, turmeric, cinnamon, cardamom pods, star anise and bay leaves in a saucepan with 3 cups of water. Stir well and bring to a boil. Reduce the heat, cover and simmer gently for 50–60 minutes, or until the liquid is absorbed. Remove the whole spices. Transfer the mixture to a large bowl. Whisk 2 tablespoons of the oil with the lemon juice, then fork through the rice mixture.

Steam or boil the broccoli and carrots until tender. Drain and refresh in cold water.

Heat the remaining oil in a large frying pan and add the onion, garlic and pepper. Stir-fry for 2–3 minutes, then add the garam masala and coriander and stir-fry for a further 1–2 minutes. Add the cooked vegetables and peas and toss to coat in the spice mixture. Add to the rice and fork through to combine. Cover and refrigerate until cold.

To make the dressing, mix the yogurt, lemon juice, mint and cumin seeds together, then season with freshly ground black pepper. Spoon the salad into six individual bowls or onto a platter and top with the dressing.

nutrition per serving: Energy 388 Cal; Fat 11.9 g; Saturated fat 2.0 g; Protein 17.1 g; Carbohydrate 48.1 g; Fiber 10.5 g; Cholesterol 7 mg

TUNA, WHITE BEAN AND TOMATO SALAD

READY IN UNDER 30 MINUTES, THIS MEAL IS A GOOD CHOICE FOR A QUICK AND HEALTHY WEEKDAY DINNER. SERVE WITH WHOLEGRAIN BREAD FOR A COMPLETE, SATISFYING MEAL.

3 eggs
1 lb 14 oz canned tuna in spring water, drained
1 garlic clove, crushed
1 tbsp roughly chopped thyme
1 tbsp finely chopped flat-leaf (Italian) parsley
½ cup fat-free, low-calorie Italian dressing

14 oz canned cannellini beans, drained and rinsed
1 large red onion, coarsely chopped
3 ripe tomatoes, cut into wedges

PREP TIME: 20 MINUTES
COOKING TIME: 5 MINUTES
SERVINGS: 4–6

Fill a saucepan with cold water and gently add the eggs. Bring to a boil, then reduce the heat and simmer for 6 minutes. Drain and plunge the eggs into cold water to stop the cooking process. Peel and cut into wedges.

Drain the tuna and flake into chunks. Combine the garlic, thyme, parsley and dressing in a bowl and whisk with a fork. Season with freshly ground black pepper.

Combine the beans and onion in a large bowl, add the dressing and toss well. Add the tuna, toss gently, then add half the egg wedges and half the tomato. Lightly combine. Pile on a platter and garnish with the remaining egg and tomato.

nutrition per serving (6): Energy 230 Cal; Fat 5.6 g; Saturated fat 1.9 g; Protein 32.9 g; Carbohydrate 9.3 g; Fiber 4.5; Cholesterol 160 mg

THIS IS A NUTRITIOUS AND SATISFYING VEGETARIAN MEAL OR SIDE DISH. IT IS LOW IN FAT AND RICH IN BETACAROTENE, FIBER AND POTASSIUM.

nutrition per serving (6): Energy 180 Cal
Fat 2.9 g
Saturated fat 0.3 g
Protein 8.4 g
Carbohydrate 25.4 g
Fiber 9 g
Cholesterol 0 mg

CHICKPEA AND ROAST VEGETABLE SALAD

2 medium sweet potatoes, peeled and
   cubed
2 red peppers, halved and core removed
4 slender eggplants, halved lengthways
4 zucchini, halved lengthways
4 onions, quartered
olive or canola oil spray
21 oz canned chickpeas, drained and rinsed
2 tbsp chopped flat-leaf (Italian) parsley

DRESSING
½ cup fat-free, low-calorie Italian dressing
1 garlic clove, crushed
1 tbsp chopped thyme

PREP TIME: 25 MINUTES + 30 MINUTES
   STANDING
COOKING TIME: 40 MINUTES
SERVINGS: 8

Preheat the oven to 425°F. Line two baking trays with baking paper and lay out the vegetables in a single layer. Lightly spray with oil.

Bake for 40 minutes, or until the vegetables are tender and begin to brown slightly on the edges. Allow to cool. Remove the skins from the pepper if you like. Chop the pepper, eggplant and zucchini into pieces, then put the vegetables in a bowl with the chickpeas and half the parsley.

Whisk together the dressing ingredients. Season with freshly ground black pepper, then toss with the vegetables. Leave for 30 minutes, then sprinkle with the rest of the parsley before serving.

WARM MARINATED MUSHROOM SALAD

THIS TASTY SALAD IS A GREAT SIDE DISH AT BARBECUES. IT IS LOW GI AND A GOOD SOURCE OF ANTIOXIDANTS.

1½ lbs mixed mushrooms
  (see Hint)
2 garlic cloves, finely chopped
½ tsp green peppercorns, crushed
2 tbsp olive oil
4 tbsp freshly squeezed orange juice
¼ cup salad leaves, such as lettuce,
  arugula, watercress or baby spinach
  leaves

olive or canola oil spray
1 tsp finely grated orange zest

PREP TIME: 25 MINUTES + 20 MINUTES
  MARINATING
COOKING TIME: 5 MINUTES
SERVINGS: 4

Trim the mushroom stems and wipe the mushrooms with a damp paper towel. Cut any large mushrooms in half. Mix together the garlic, peppercorns, olive oil and orange juice. Pour over the mushrooms and marinate for about 20 minutes.

Arrange the salad leaves in a dish.

Heat a cast-iron skillet to hot. Spray with oil. Drain the mushrooms, reserving the marinade. First cook the flat and button mushrooms on the pan for about 2 minutes. Add the softer mushrooms and cook for 1 minute, or until they just soften.

Scatter the mushrooms over the salad leaves and drizzle with the marinade. Sprinkle with orange zest and season well with freshly ground black pepper.

HINT:
• Try a mix of mushrooms, such as baby button, oyster, Swiss brown, shiitake and enoki.

nutrition per serving: Energy 164 Cal; Fat 10.3 g; Saturated fat 1.4 g; Protein 7.6 g; Carbohydrate 6.6 g; Fiber 6.5 g; Cholesterol 0 mg

SALAD NIÇOISE

THIS COLORFUL AND NUTRITIOUS SALAD, A MEDITERRANEAN FAVORITE, IS AN EXCELLENT WAY TO INCLUDE THE NUTRITIONAL BENEFITS OF FISH IN YOUR DIET.

4 eggs

1 cup green beans, trimmed

6 artichoke hearts in brine, drained

12 oz mixed salad leaves

4 tomatoes, cut into wedges

15 oz canned tuna in spring water, drained and separated into chunks

1 red pepper, cut into strips

14 oz canned cannellini beans, drained and rinsed

1 tbsp capers

10 small black olives

1 tbsp chopped tarragon

DRESSING

1 garlic clove, crushed

3 tsp Dijon mustard

2 anchovy fillets in brine, drained and finely chopped

½ cup fat-free, low-calorie French dressing

PREP TIME: 25 MINUTES

COOKING TIME: 10 MINUTES

SERVINGS: 4–6

Fill a saucepan with cold water and gently add the eggs. Bring to a boil, then reduce the heat and simmer for 6 minutes. Drain and plunge the eggs into cold water to stop the cooking process. Peel and cut into wedges.

Put the beans in a saucepan of boiling water, return to a boil for 2 minutes, then drain and rinse under cold water. Chill in a bowl of iced water. Cut the artichokes into halves or quarters.

Arrange the salad leaves on a platter or individual plates. Top with the green beans, tomato, artichoke, tuna, egg, red pepper and cannellini beans. Sprinkle with the capers and olives.

To make the dressing, put the garlic, mustard, anchovies and dressing in a bowl and whisk until well blended. Season with freshly ground black pepper and drizzle over the salad. Sprinkle with tarragon.

nutrition per serving (6): Energy 223 Cal; Fat 6.2 g; Saturated fat 1.7 g; Protein 24.8 g; Carbohydrate 12.4 g; Fiber 8.5 g; Cholesterol 170 mg

WARM LAMB SALAD

2 tbsp red curry paste

3 tbsp chopped cilantro leaves

1 tbsp finely grated fresh ginger

1 tbsp peanut oil

1½ to 2 lbs lean lamb loin fillets, trimmed
   and thinly sliced

7 oz snow peas, trimmed

1 lb 5 oz thick fresh rice noodles

olive or canola oil spray

1 red pepper, thinly sliced

1 cucumber, thinly sliced

6 spring onions (scallions), thinly sliced

DRESSING

1 tbsp peanut oil

3 tbsp lime juice

2 tsp brown sugar

3 tsp fish sauce

3 tsp reduced-sodium soy sauce

4 tbsp chopped mint leaves

1 garlic clove, crushed

PREP TIME: 30 MINUTES + 3 HOURS
   REFRIGERATION

COOKING TIME: 15 MINUTES

SERVINGS: 4–6

Combine the curry paste, cilantro, ginger and peanut oil in a bowl. Add the lamb and coat well. Cover and refrigerate for 2–3 hours.

Steam or boil the snow peas until just tender, then refresh under cold water and drain.

Put the noodles in a large heatproof bowl, cover with boiling water and soak for 8 minutes, or until softened. Separate gently and drain.

To make the dressing, put all the ingredients in a small bowl and whisk until well blended.

Heat a wok until very hot. Spray with the oil. Add half the lamb and stir-fry for 5 minutes, or until tender. Repeat with the remaining lamb, using more spray oil if needed.

Put the lamb, snow peas, noodles, pepper, cucumber and spring onion in a large bowl, drizzle with the dressing and toss together before serving

HINT:
• This recipe can also be made into a gluten-free version if you use gluten-free fish sauce and gluten-free soy sauce.

THIS SALAD IS A GOOD SOURCE
OF IRON, ZINC AND
ANTIOXIDANTS.

nutrition per serving (6): Energy 435 Cal
Fat 12.6 g
Saturated fat 3.2 g
Protein 31.8 g
Carbohydrate 46.2 g
Fiber 3 g
Cholesterol 81 mg

TOFU SALAD WITH GINGER MISO DRESSING

THIS ASIAN-THEMED SALAD IS A DELICIOUS, LIGHT, VEGETARIAN MEAL OR SIDE DISH. SERVE WITH FRESH RICE NOODLES OR BASMATI RICE.

4½ tbsp tamari (see Hint)
1 tsp olive or canola oil
2 garlic cloves, crushed
1 tsp grated fresh ginger
1 tsp chili paste
1 lb firm tofu, cut into
   small cubes
14 oz mixed Asian salad leaves
1 cucumber, thinly sliced
9 oz cherry tomatoes, halved
olive or canola oil spray

DRESSING
2 tsp white miso paste
2 tbsp mirin
1 tsp sesame oil
1 tsp grated fresh ginger
1 tsp finely chopped chives
1 tbsp sesame seeds, toasted

PREP TIME: 20 MINUTES + 10 MINUTES
   MARINATING
COOKING TIME: 5 MINUTES
SERVINGS: 4

Mix together the tamari, oil, garlic, ginger and chili paste in a bowl. Add the tofu and mix well. Marinate for 10 minutes. Drain, reserving the marinade.

Put the salad leaves, cucumber and tomato in a bowl.

To make the dressing, combine the miso with ½ cup hot water and leave until the miso dissolves. Add the mirin, sesame oil, ginger, chives and sesame seeds and stir until it begins to thicken.

Heat a cast-iron skillet to hot. Spray with oil. Add the tofu and cook over medium heat for 4 minutes, or until golden brown. Increase the heat to high, pour on the reserved marinade and cook for a further 1 minute over high heat. Cool for 5 minutes.

Add the tofu to the salad, drizzle with the dressing and toss well.

HINT:
• Tamari is a naturally fermented, thick, dark Japanese soy sauce. You can use reduced-sodium soy sauce instead.

nutrition per serving: Energy 255 Cal; Fat 13.2 g; Saturated fat 1.9 g; Protein 19.8 g; Carbohydrate 11.2 g; Fiber 6.2 g; Cholesterol 0 mg

TABOULEH

THIS POPULAR SALAD IS VERY VERSATILE—SERVE IT WITH MEAT OR FISH, USE IT IN A SANDWICH OR EAT IT ON ITS OWN. IF YOU LIKE TO EXPERIMENT, LOOK FOR CRACKED BARLEY IN HEALTH FOOD SHOPS TO USE AS A SUBSTITUTE FOR THE BULGUR.

¾ cup bulgur

2 bunches (about 10½ oz) flat-leaf (Italian) parsley

1 handful mint leaves

4 spring onions (scallions), finely chopped

4 tomatoes, finely chopped

2 garlic cloves, crushed

3 tbsp lemon juice

2 tbsp olive oil

PREP TIME: 20 MINUTES + 15 MINUTES STANDING

COOKING TIME: NONE

SERVINGS: 6–8

Put the bulgur in a bowl with 3¼ cups of water and leave for 15 minutes, or until all the water has been absorbed.

Finely chop the herbs with a large sharp knife or in a food processor. Take care not to over-process.

Put the bulgur, herbs, spring onion, tomato, garlic, lemon juice and oil in a bowl and toss well. Refrigerate until required. Return to room temperature to serve.

nutrition per serving (8): Energy 120 Cal; Fat 5 g; Saturated fat 0.7 g; Protein 3.7 g; Carbohydrate 11.4 g; Fiber 6.0 g; Cholesterol 0 mg

A LOW-GI DISH WITH A TANGY FLAVOR, THIS SALAD PROVIDES ANTIOXIDANTS, FOLATE, IRON AND ZINC—SUITABLE AS A LIGHT MEAL OR A QUICKLY PREPARED DINNER.

nutrition per serving: Energy 418 Cal
Fat 7.4 g
Saturated fat 2.6 g
Protein 34.1 g
Carbohydrate 50.6 g
Fiber 3.7 g
Cholesterol 80 mg

MINTY BEEF NOODLE SALAD

olive or canola oil spray

about 1 lb piece lean beef rump
    steak

9 oz dry thin rice vermicelli
    noodles

9 oz cherry tomatoes, halved

7 oz baby Asian salad leaves

1 cucumber, peeled, seeded and thinly
    sliced

¼ red onion, cut into thin slivers

6 radishes, thinly sliced

1 handful mint

DRESSING

3 tbsp lime juice

3 tbsp reduced-sodium soy sauce

2 tbsp fish sauce

2 tbsp grated palm sugar or brown sugar

2 small red chilies, seeded and finely
    chopped

PREP TIME: 20 MINUTES

COOKING TIME: 10 MINUTES

SERVINGS: 4

Heat a large, non-stick frying pan and spray with the oil. Pat the meat dry with paper towels. Season well with freshly ground black pepper. Put the meat in the pan and brown on both sides. Cook for a further 5–8 minutes, or until cooked as desired. Cover with foil and set aside for 5 minutes, then cut into thin slices.

Combine the dressing ingredients in a small bowl, stirring to dissolve the sugar.

Cover the noodles with boiling water and set aside for 5 minutes, or until softened. Drain and cool. Use scissors to cut into smaller lengths.

Combine the cherry tomatoes, salad greens, cucumber, onion, radishes and mint leaves in a large bowl. Toss through the noodles and beef, then pour over the dressing.

SPICY THAI PORK SALAD

THIS SPICY SALAD GETS TOP MARKS FOR GOOD TASTE AND HAS THE ADDED BENEFITS OF BEING HEART HEALTHY AND QUICK TO MAKE. SERVE WITH FRESH RICE NOODLES, MUNG BEAN NOODLES OR BASMATI RICE FOR A COMPLETE LOW-GI MEAL.

⅓ cup raw unsalted peanuts

2 tsp olive or canola oil

2 stems lemon grass, white part only, thinly sliced

2 green chilies, finely chopped

about 1 lb lean ground pork

2 tsp finely grated lime zest

3 tbsp lime juice

2–6 tsp chili sauce

lettuce leaves, to serve

1 handful cilantro leaves

1 small handful small mint leaves

1 small onion, very finely sliced

3 tbsp chopped fresh shallots

PREP TIME: 20 MINUTES

COOKING TIME: 10 MINUTES

SERVINGS: 4–6

Preheat the oven to 350°F. Put the peanuts on a baking tray. Cook for 5 minutes, stirring once, until the peanuts are lightly golden. Cool then chop.

Heat a wok until very hot, add the oil and swirl to coat. Add the lemon grass, chili and pork. Stir-fry, breaking up any lumps with a fork or wooden spoon, over high heat for 6 minutes, or until cooked through. Transfer to a bowl and set aside to cool completely.

Add the lime zest, lime juice, and the chili sauce to taste, to the cooled pork mixture. Arrange the lettuce leaves on a plate. Stir most of the cilantro and mint leaves, onion, peanuts and shallots through the pork mixture. Spoon over the lettuce and sprinkle the rest of the mint leaves, onion, peanuts and shallots over the top to serve.

nutrition per serving (6): Energy 195 Cal; Fat 11.5 g; Saturated fat 2.9 g; Protein 19.2 g; Carbohydrate 2.7 g; Fiber 1.3 g; Cholesterol 50 mg

HOT BEAN SALAD

A SATISFYING COMBINATION OF HIGH-FIBER BEANS AND NUTRITIOUS VEGETABLES AND HERBS, RICH IN SLOW-RELEASE CARBOHYDRATE AND SOLUBLE FIBER, THIS SALAD IS IDEAL IF YOU ARE WATCHING YOUR BLOOD SUGAR AND CHOLESTEROL LEVELS.

¼ cup dried chickpeas
¼ cup dried pinto beans
¼ cup dried red kidney beans
¼ cup dried black-eyed beans
1 tbsp olive or canola oil
2 onions, sliced
2 tsp ground cumin
1 tsp ground coriander
15 oz canned corn kernels, drained
2 tomatoes, chopped

4 tbsp lemon juice
1 large handful cilantro leaves, chopped
1 cucumber, grated
1 cup low-fat plain yogurt

PREP TIME: 15 MINUTES + OVERNIGHT
  SOAKING
COOKING TIME: 1 HOUR 15 MINUTES
SERVINGS: 8

Combine the chickpeas, pinto beans, red kidney beans and black-eyed beans in a large bowl. Cover with water and soak overnight. Drain, place in a large saucepan and cover with water. Bring to a boil, then reduce the heat and simmer for 45 minutes, or until tender. Don't overcook or the beans will be mushy.

Meanwhile, in a large, deep non-stick frying pan, heat the oil and then add the onion. Cook over low heat for 25 minutes, or until golden. Add the cumin and coriander with the beans, and toss to combine. Add the corn kernels, tomato, lemon juice and cilantro. Season with freshly ground black pepper and stir.

Squeeze out the moisture from the cucumber. Combine the cucumber with the yogurt, and season. Stir to combine.

Put the hot bean mixture on a serving plate, and top with the yogurt mixture.

nutrition per serving: Energy 229 Cal; Fat 2.3 g; Saturated fat 0.3 g; Protein 14.7 g; Carbohydrate 31.7 g; Fiber 11.4 g; Cholesterol 2 mg

MAIN MEALS

TOFU WITH GREENS AND NOODLES

MARINADE
3 tbsp oyster sauce
3 tbsp hoisin sauce
2 tbsp reduced-sodium soy sauce
1½ tbsp brown sugar
3 tsp grated ginger
3 garlic cloves, crushed

10½ oz firm tofu, drained and
cut into ¾ in cubes
10½ oz dried thin egg noodles
1 tsp olive or canola oil
4 Asian shallots, thinly sliced

1 small red pepper, seeded and thinly
sliced
7 oz sugar snap peas, trimmed
14 oz broccolini, cut into 2 in lengths (see
Hint)
½ cup reduced-salt vegetable stock
cilantro leaves, to serve

PREP TIME: 15 MINUTES + 30 MINUTES
MARINATING
COOKING TIME: 15 MINUTES
SERVINGS: 4

Combine the marinade ingredients in a non-metallic bowl. Add the tofu and gently stir through. Cover and refrigerate for at least 30 minutes, longer if possible.

Cook the noodles according to the manufacturer's directions and drain. Cut the noodles into shorter lengths using scissors.

Heat the oil in a large wok. Add the shallots and pepper and stir-fry for 2 minutes, or until slightly softened. Add the peas, broccolini and stock. Cover and cook for 2–3 minutes, or until the vegetables are just tender, stirring occasionally.

Add the tofu with the marinade ingredients and the noodles. Gently combine and stir until heated through. Serve immediately garnished with the coriander leaves.

HINT:
• Use broccoli florets if broccolini is not available.

IF YOU THINK TOFU IS BLAND, YOU NEED TO TRY THIS DISH. WHEN MARINATED, THE TOFU SOAKS UP ALL THE FLAVORS. THIS DISH IS A GOOD SOURCE OF ANTIOXIDANTS, FOLATE, FIBER AND IRON.

nutrition per serving: Energy 508 Cal
Fat 9 g
Saturated fat 1.3 g
Protein 26.4 g
Carbohydrate 73.2 g
Fiber 11.1 g
Cholesterol 14 mg

THAI CHICKEN AND HOLY BASIL STIR-FRY

THIS LOW-GI AROMATIC THAI MEAL PROVIDES GOOD AMOUNTS OF MOST VITAMINS AND MINERALS. THE FRESH FLAVORS ARE PERFECT TO ENJOY ON A SUMMER NIGHT.

14 oz fresh rice noodles

3 tbsp fish sauce

3 tbsp lime juice

1 tomato, diced

2 handfuls Thai basil

about 1 lb skinless chicken breast fillets

2 tsp olive or canola oil

3 garlic cloves, thinly sliced

4 spring onions (scallions), thinly sliced

2 small red chilies, seeded and thinly sliced

1 cup snow peas, trimmed

PREP TIME: 15 MINUTES

COOKING TIME: 20 MINUTES

SERVINGS: 4

Put the rice noodles in a large heatproof bowl. Cover with boiling water and soak for 8 minutes, or until softened. Seperate gently and drain. Use scissors to cut into shorter lengths.

Meanwhile, to make the stir-fry sauce, put the fish sauce, lime juice, tomato, basil and 1 tablespoon water in a small bowl and mix well.

Trim the chicken and thinly slice. Heat a wok over high heat, add the oil and swirl to coat. Add the garlic, spring onion and chili and stir-fry for 1 minute, or until fragrant. Add the chicken in small batches and stir-fry for 3 minutes, or until lightly browned. Remove from the wok and set aside. Reheat the wok between batches.

Return all the chicken to the wok. Add the snow peas and stir-fry sauce to the wok and scrape any sediment from the bottom. Stir through the noodles. Reduce the heat and simmer for 2 minutes, or until the tomato is soft and the chicken cooked through. Serve immediately.

nutrition per serving: Energy 432 Cal; Fat 10.3 g; Saturated fat 2.3 g; Protein 34.8 g; Carbohydrate 46.7 g; Fiber 4.1 g; Cholesterol 82 mg

TERIYAKI PORK WITH STEAMED ASIAN GREENS

THIS POPULAR ASIAN DISH IS LOW IN FAT AND A RICH SOURCE OF PROTEIN, ANTIOXIDANTS, FOLATE AND POTASSIUM.

about 1 lb lean pork fillet
½ cup reduced-sodium soy sauce
½ cup mirin
½ cup unsweetened apple juice
1 tbsp grated ginger
1¼ in x 1¼ in piece ginger, sliced
1 bunch (about 10½ oz) Chinese broccoli,
  cut into 4 in lengths
7 oz asparagus, trimmed and cut into 2 in
  pieces
4 oz canned baby corn, trimmed
1 tsp sesame oil

olive or canola oil spray
basmati or doongara rice, to serve
  (see Hint)

PREP TIME: 20 MINUTES + 1 HOUR
  MARINATING
COOKING TIME: 20 MINUTES
SERVINGS: 4

Thinly slice the pork across the grain. Mix the soy, mirin, apple juice and ginger in a large, non-metallic bowl. Add the pork and toss to coat well. Cover and refrigerate for 1 hour.

Meanwhile, fill a wok one-third full of water, and bring to a simmer over a low heat. Line the base of a bamboo steamer with the ginger slices and top with the broccoli, asparagus and corn. Cover with the lid, place over the wok, making sure the water doesn't touch the base, and steam for 5–6 minutes, or until the vegetables are just cooked. Discard the ginger, drizzle with the sesame oil and season with pepper.

At the same time, lightly spray a non-stick wok with oil and heat over a high heat. Add the pork in two batches and cook for 2–3 minutes, or until cooked. Set aside. Add the marinade and simmer for 4–5 minutes, or until reduced and thickened. Return the pork and stir until warmed through. Serve with the steamed vegetables and rice.

HINT:
• The rice will add a lot more carbohydrate, so if you have difficulty controlling your blood sugar level make sure that you have no more than 1 cup of cooked rice.

nutrition per serving: Energy 296 Cal; Fat 5.1 g; Saturated fat 1.2 g; Protein 33.1 g; Carbohydrate 23.8 g; Fiber 4.5 g; Cholesterol 119 mg

THIS LOW-GI, HIGH-PROTEIN DISH IS A GOOD SOURCE OF B-GROUP VITAMINS, POTASSIUM AND PHOSPHORUS. IT'S A GREAT CHOICE FOR THOSE WATCHING THEIR WEIGHT.

nutrition per serving: Energy 408 Cal
Fat 6.2 g
Saturated fat 1.1 g
Protein 49.1 g
Carbohydrate 45.7 g
Fiber 4.9 g
Cholesterol 83 mg

RICE NOODLES WITH FISH AND BLACK BEANS

14 oz fresh rice noodles

1 small bunch (about 7 oz) Chinese broccoli, cut into 2 in lengths

2 tbsp reduced-sodium soy sauce

1½ tbsp Chinese rice wine (optional)

½ tsp sesame oil

1 tsp cornstarch

about 1 lb skinless snapper or blue eye fillets

2 tsp olive or canola oil

5 garlic cloves, crushed

2 tsp finely chopped ginger

2 spring onions (scallions), finely chopped, plus extra, thinly sliced on the diagonal, to garnish

2 small red chilies, finely chopped

2 tbsp canned salted black beans, rinsed, roughly chopped

⅔ cup reduced-salt fish or vegetable stock

PREP TIME: 20 MINUTES

COOKING TIME: 20 MINUTES

SERVINGS: 4

Put the noodles in a large heatproof bowl, cover with boiling water and soak for 8 minutes, or until softened. Separate gently and drain.

Put the Chinese broccoli in a steamer, cover and steam over a wok or large saucepan of simmering water for 2 minutes, or until slightly wilted. Remove from the heat and keep warm.

To make the marinade, combine the soy sauce, rice wine, sesame oil and cornstarch in a large non-metallic bowl. Cut the fish into 1½ in pieces, checking for bones. Add to the marinade and toss to coat well.

Heat a wok over high heat, add the oil and swirl to coat. Add the garlic, ginger, spring onion, chili and black beans and stir-fry for 1 minute. Add the fish and marinade and cook for 2 minutes, or until the fish is almost cooked through. Remove the fish with a slotted spoon and keep warm. Add the stock to the wok and bring to a boil. Reduce the heat to low and bring to a simmer. Cook for 5 minutes, or until the sauce has slightly thickened. Return the fish to the wok, cover with a lid and simmer gently for 2–3 minutes, or until just cooked.

Divide the noodles among four plates, top with the Chinese broccoli and spoon the fish and black bean sauce on top. Garnish with the extra spring onion.

DIABETES

BEEF SKEWERS WITH TOMATO MINT SALAD

THIS MEAL IS QUICK AND EASY TO MAKE AND IS LOADED WITH FOLATE, POTASSIUM AND ANTIOXIDANTS.

about 1½ lbs lean beef sirloin steaks
1 large red pepper
8 x 1¾ in flat or button mushrooms

MARINADE
3 tbsp reduced-salt teriyaki sauce
1 tbsp honey
1 tbsp lemon juice
2 garlic cloves, crushed

TOMATO MINT SALAD
4 vine-ripened tomatoes, seeded and
  chopped
3 spring onions (scallions), chopped

1 cucumber, seeded and chopped
2 handfuls mint, chopped
2 tbsp fat-free, low-calorie Italian dressing

olive or canola oil spray
1 tbsp sesame seeds, toasted
basmati or doongara rice, to serve
  (see Hint)

PREP TIME: 25 MINUTES + SOAKING AND
  MARINATING TIME
COOKING TIME: 25 MINUTES
SERVINGS: 4

Soak 8 long, wooden skewers in water for 15 minutes. Cut the meat into bite-sized cubes. Seed the pepper, then cut into 1¼ in cubes. Thread the meat onto the skewers, alternating with the mushrooms and pepper.

Combine the marinade ingredients in a non-metallic flat dish. Lay the skewers in the marinade and coat well. Refrigerate for at least 20 minutes, turning occasionally.

Combine the tomato mint salad ingredients in a bowl.

Meanwhile, preheat a broiler or barbecue. Cook the mainated skewers, turning and spraying lightly with the oil, for 8 minutes, or until just cooked. Brush 2 or 3 times with the remaining marinade. Scatter over the sesame seeds. Serve the skewers with the tomato mint salad and rice.

HINT:
• The rice will add a lot more carbohydrate, so if you have difficulty controlling your blood sugar level make sure that you have no more than 1 cup of cooked rice.

nutrition per serving: Energy 335 Cal; Fat 12.3 g; Saturated fat 4.4 g; Protein 37.6 g; Carbohydrate 15.3 g; Fiber 5.5 g; Cholesterol 87 mg

FRIED RICE

A REDUCED-FAT FRIED RICE, THIS VERSION IS HIGH IN PROTEIN AND CARBOHYDRATE, WITH GOOD AMOUNTS OF VITAMIN C, B-GROUP VITAMINS, POTASSIUM AND PHOSPHORUS.

olive or canola oil spray
4 egg whites, lightly beaten
2 garlic cloves, crushed
12 oz raw shrimp, peeled, deveined and halved lengthways
3½ oz cooked skinless chicken, shredded
½ cup frozen peas
6½ oz sliced light ham, cut into small strips
1 red pepper, diced
4 spring onions (scallions), sliced

4 cups cooked basmati or basmati wild rice (see Hint)
1½ tbsp sodium-reduced soy sauce
3 tsp fish sauce
1½ tsp brown sugar

PREP TIME: 20 MINUTES
COOKING TIME: 15 MINUTES
SERVINGS: 6

Lightly spray a non-stick wok with oil and pour in the egg white. Cook over low heat, stirring until the egg is just cooked and slightly scrambled, then remove and set aside.

Add the garlic, shrimp, chicken, peas, ham and pepper to the wok, and stir-fry for 3–4 minutes, or until the shrimp are cooked.

Add the spring onion, rice, soy sauce, fish sauce and sugar, and toss for 30 seconds, or until heated through. Add the egg, toss lightly and serve.

HINT:
• You will need to cook 1⅓ cups rice blend for this recipe.

nutrition per serving: Energy 293 Cal; Fat 3.4 g; Saturated fat 0.9 g; Protein 24.6 g; Carbohydrate 38.2 g; Fiber 1.8 g; Cholesterol 85 mg

SPICY CHICKEN STIR-FRY

4 dried shiitake mushrooms

9 oz fresh rice noodles or dried mung bean noodles

olive or canola oil spray

1 red onion, cut into thin wedges

2 garlic cloves, crushed

¾ in x ¾ in piece fresh ginger, julienned

1 tbsp chili jam

about 1 lb skinless chicken breast fillet, cut into strips

½ red pepper, cut into thin strips

about 2 lbs Chinese broccoli, cut into 2 in lengths

4 oz canned baby corn, halved on the diagonal

1½ cups snowpeas, halved on the diagonal

4 tbsp reduced-sodium soy sauce

2 tbsp mirin

1 large handful cilantro leaves

PREP TIME: 20 MINUTES + 15 MINUTES SOAKING

COOKING TIME: 15 MINUTES

SERVINGS: 4

Place the mushrooms in a heatproof bowl and cover with 1½ cups boiling water and stand for 15 minutes. Drain, reserving the liquid and squeezing out any excess liquid. Remove the stalks and thinly slice the caps. Place the noodles in a heatproof bowl, pour over boiling water to cover and stand for 5 minutes, or until tender. Drain.

Meanwhile, heat a non-stick wok over a high heat and spray with the oil. Add the onion and cook for 2–3 minutes. Add the garlic, ginger and chili jam and cook for a further 1 minute, adding 1–2 tablespoons of the reserved mushroom liquid to mix in the chili jam.

Add the chicken and cook for 4–5 minutes, or until almost cooked through. Add the pepper, broccoli, corn, snowpeas, mushrooms and 3 tablespoons reserved mushroom liquid and stir-fry for 2–3 minutes, or until the vegetables are tender. Add the soy sauce, mirin, cilantro and noodles and season with ground white pepper. Toss until well combined and serve immediately.

HINT:
• Dried shiitake mushrooms, chili jam and mirin are readily available in supermarkets and Asian food stores.

STIR-FRIES ARE AN EASY WAY
TO INCLUDE MORE VEGETABLES
IN YOUR DIET. THIS PEPPED-UP, TASTY
DISH OFFERS GOOD AMOUNTS OF
ANTIOXIDANTS, B-GROUP VITAMINS
AND IRON.

nutrition per serving: Energy 360 Cal

Fat 7.3 g

Saturated fat 1.8 g

Protein 32.2 g

Carbohydrate 34.8 g

Fiber 11.3 g

Cholesterol 66 mg

STIR-FRIED THAI BEEF

APART FROM THE MARINATING TIME, THIS DISH IS QUICK TO MAKE AND IS A GOOD CHOICE FOR BUSY PEOPLE. IT CONTAINS ANTIOXIDANTS, FOLATE, IRON AND ZINC.

about 1 lb lean sirloin steak, trimmed
2–3 bird's eye chilies, seeded and finely chopped
3 garlic cloves, crushed
1 tsp palm sugar or brown sugar
2 tbsp fish sauce
2 tsp olive or canola oil
1 cup yard-long or green beans, sliced into 1¼ in lengths
1 cup sugar snap peas, trimmed
1 large carrot, thinly sliced

1 large handful Thai basil
1–2 bird's eye chilies, seeded and finely sliced (optional), to garnish
basmati or doongara rice, to serve (see Hints)

PREP TIME: 15 MINUTES + 2 HOURS MARINATING
COOKING TIME: 25 MINUTES
SERVINGS: 4

Slice the meat as thinly as possible, cutting across the grain. Place in a non-metallic bowl with the chili, garlic, palm sugar, fish sauce and 1 teaspoon of the oil. Toss well to combine, cover and refrigerate for 2 hours.

Blanch the beans, sugar snap peas and carrot in a large saucepan of boiling water for 2 minutes, drain and refresh. Heat the remaining oil in a large, non-stick wok until very hot and stir-fry the beef in 2 batches over high heat until just browned.

Return all the beef to the wok with the blanched vegetables and basil. Stir-fry for a further 1–2 minutes, or until warmed through. Garnish with sliced chilies, if you like, and serve with the rice.

HINTS:
- To save time in the evening, you can prepare the meat in the morning and leave it in the fridge to marinate during the day.
- The rice will add a lot more carbohydrate, so if you have difficulty controlling your blood sugar level make sure that you have no more than 1 cup of cooked rice.

nutrition per serving: Energy 211 Cal; Fat 8.9 g; Saturated fat 2.9 g; Protein 24.4 g; Carbohydrate 5.8 g; Fiber 4.2 g; Cholesterol 58 mg

TANDOORI PORK KEBABS

THE INDIAN SPICES BLEND BEAUTIFULLY WITH THE PORK TO PRODUCE A MEAL THAT'S RICH IN FLAVOR. THIS DISH IS A GOOD SOURCE OF PROTEIN, POTASSIUM AND PHOSPHORUS.

1 cup low-fat plain yogurt
2 garlic cloves, crushed
2 tbsp tandoori paste
1 tbsp lemon juice
2 tbsp chopped cilantro leaves
about 1½ lbs lean pork fillet, cubed
1 tsp olive or canola oil
1 onion, chopped
2 garlic cloves, crushed, extra
2 tsp ground cumin
½ tsp paprika
1 tsp ground coriander

2 cups basmati rice
4 cups reduced-salt vegetable stock
¾ cup low-fat plain yogurt, extra
1 tbsp chopped cilantro leaves, extra

PREP TIME: 20 MINUTES + 4 HOURS
   MARINATING
COOKING TIME: 40 MINUTES
SERVINGS: 4

Combine the yogurt, garlic, tandoori paste, lemon juice and cilantro in a large, non-metallic bowl. Add the pork and stir to coat. Refrigerate, covered, for 4 hours.

Heat the oil in a heavy-based saucepan, add the onion, garlic, spices and coriander and cook for 5 minutes, or until golden. Add the rice and stir to coat. Add the stock, bring to a boil, then simmer for 10 minutes, or until tunnels appear in the rice. Reduce the heat to low, cover and cook for 10 minutes.

Thread the pork onto 8 skewers. Heat a cast-iron skillet and cook for 3–5 minutes on each side, or until tender.

Combine the extra yogurt and cilantro and serve with the pork and spiced rice. Serve with a salad.

HINT:
• Marinate the pork in the morning before work, then cook when you get home.

nutrition per serving: Energy 634 Cal; Fat 6.8 g; Saturated fat 1.9 g; Protein 48 g; Carbohydrate 91.5 g; Fiber 4.6 g; Cholesterol 168 mg

THIS CLASSIC THAI DISH IS A GREAT
CHOICE FOR WEIGHT WATCHERS. IT IS A
FILLING VEGETARIAN MEAL AND MAKES
DELICIOUS LEFTOVERS.

nutrition per serving (6): Energy 272 Cal
Fat 6.9 g
Saturated fat 3.2 g
Protein 6.2 g
Carbohydrate 42.3 g
Fiber 9.2 g
Cholesterol 0 mg

GREEN VEGETABLE CURRY WITH BARLEY

1½ cups pearl barley

2 tsp olive or canola oil

1 onion, chopped

1–2 tbsp green curry paste

1 eggplant, cut into quarters and sliced

1½ cups light coconut milk

1 cup reduced-salt vegetable stock

6 kaffir lime leaves

1 sweet potato, peeled and cut into cubes

1 tsp brown sugar

2 tbsp lime juice

2 tsp grated lime zest

basmati or doongar rice, to serve
  (see Hints)

PREP TIME: 15 MINUTES

COOKING TIME: 55 MINUTES

SERVINGS: 4–6

Rinse and drain the barley. Put in a large saucepan with 5 cups water. Bring to a boil, then reduce the heat and simmer for 25–30 minutes, or until tender. Drain.

Meanwhile, heat the oil in a large wok or frying pan. Add the onion and curry paste and cook, stirring, over medium heat for 3 minutes. Add the eggplant and cook for a further 4–5 minutes, or until softened.

Pour in the coconut milk and stock, bring to a boil, then reduce the heat and simmer for 5 minutes. Add the kaffir lime leaves and sweet potato and cook for 10 minutes, or until the eggplant and sweet potato are very tender.

Mix in the sugar, lime juice and lime zest until well combined with the vegetables. Season to taste with freshly ground black pepper and serve with the barley.

HINTS:
- Strict vegetarians should be sure to read the label and choose a green curry paste that doesn't contain shrimp paste. Alternatively, make your own curry pastes.
- The rice will add more carbohydrate, so choose a small serving.

LAMB KEBABS, RAITA AND BULGUR SALAD

NOT ONLY DOES THIS MEAL TASTE DELICIOUS, IT IS ALSO RICH IN CARBOHYDRATE AND PROTEIN AND IS A GOOD SOURCE OF MANY VITAMINS AND MINERALS.

LAMB KEBABS
1 to 1½ lbs lean lamb
1 tbsp Moroccan seasoning
2 tsp lemon juice
2 garlic cloves, crushed

RAITA
1½ cups low-fat plain yogurt
1 small cucumber, peeled, seeded and
  diced
1 large handful mint, chopped

BULGUR SALAD
2 cups bulgur wheat
4½ oz cherry tomatoes, halved

1 large handful flat-leaf (Italian) parsley,
  chopped
4 tbsp chopped mint
½ cup currants
½ cup dried apricots, chopped
¼ cup pistachio nuts, chopped
2 tbsp lemon juice
2 small lemons
2 small red onions
olive or canola oil spray

PREP TIME: 20 MINUTES + MARINATING TIME
COOKING TIME: 10 MINUTES
SERVINGS: 4–6

Cut the lamb into 1¼ in cubes. Combine the Moroccan seasoning, lemon juice and garlic in a non-metallic bowl, then add the meat. Cover and refrigerate for 20 minutes.

To make the raita, combine all the ingredients in a bowl. Set aside.

Put the bulgur in a bowl and cover with warm water. Stand for 20 minutes. Drain and squeeze out excess water using clean hands. Return bulgur to bowl and stir through the tomatoes, parsley, mint, dried fruit and nuts. Drizzle with lemon juice. Set aside.

Preheat the broiler or barbecue grill. Cut each lemon into 8 wedges. Cut each onion into 8 wedges. Thread the lamb, lemon and onion wedges alternately onto 8 x 12 in metal skewers. Spray with the oil and brush with any remaining marinade. Grill or broil and turn for 10 minutes, or until the meat is cooked to your liking.

Serve the kebabs on a bed of bulgur salad and accompany with the raita.

nutrition per serving: Energy 765 Cal; Fat 13.6 g; Saturated fat 3.9 g; Protein 59.4 g; Carbohydrate 85 g; Fiber 22.9; Cholesterol 127 mg

MONGOLIAN HOTPOT

HOTPOTS ARE A GREAT WAY TO INCLUDE A VARIETY OF HEALTHY FOODS IN ONE MEAL. THIS SPICY DISH IS A GOOD SOURCE OF IRON, ZINC AND B-GROUP VITAMINS AND PROVIDES A SATISFYING LOW-GI MEAL.

14 oz fresh rice noodles

1 to 1½ lbs lean lamb backstraps or loin fillet

4 spring onions (scallions), sliced

6 cups reduced-salt chicken stock

6 thin slices ginger

2 tbsp Chinese rice wine (optional)

10½ oz silken firm tofu, cut into ⅝ in cubes

1 bunch (about 10 oz) Chinese broccoli, cut into 1½ in lengths

3 cups shredded Chinese cabbage

SAUCE

4 tbsp reduced-sodium soy sauce

2 tbsp Chinese sesame paste

1 tbsp Chinese rice wine (optional)

1 tsp chili and garlic paste

PREP TIME: 20 MINUTES

COOKING TIME: 5 MINUTES

SERVINGS: 6

Put the noodles in a large heatproof bowl. Cover with boiling water and soak for 8 minutes, or until softened. Separate gently and drain. Divide among 6 bowls.

Trim the lamb, then thinly slice across the grain. Divide the lamb strips among the bowls, then add spring onion.

Pour the stock into a 10 cup flameproof hotpot or large saucepan, then add the ginger and rice wine (if using). Cover and bring to a boil over high heat. Add the tofu, Chinese broccoli and Chinese cabbage and simmer, uncovered, for 1 minute, or until the broccoli has wilted.

To make the sauce, combine the soy sauce, sesame paste, rice wine and chili and garlic paste in a small bowl.

Divide the tofu, broccoli and cabbage among the bowls, then ladle on the hot stock—it will be hot enough to cook the lamb. Drizzle a little of the sauce on top and serve the rest on the side.

nutrition per serving: Energy 396 Cal; Fat 12.7 g; Saturated fat 3.1 g; Protein 35.8 g; Carbohydrate 32.6 g; Fiber 5.3 g; Cholesterol 65 mg

TUNA WITH LIME AND CHILI SAUCE AND GREEN VEGETABLES

SAUCE
2 large handfuls mint, chopped
2 large handfuls cilantro leaves, chopped
1 tsp grated lime zest
1 tbsp lime juice
1 tsp grated fresh ginger
1 jalapeño chili, seeded and finely chopped
1 cup low-fat plain yogurt

olive canola oil spray
4 tuna steaks
6 oz asparagus, trimmed and
    cut into 2 in pieces
½ cup snow peas, trimmed
½ cup green beans, trimmed
4 wholegrain bread rolls, to serve

PREP TIME: 20 MINUTES
COOKING TIME: 10 MINUTES
SERVINGS: 4

To make the sauce, combine the mint, cilantro, lime zest, lime juice, ginger and chili. Fold in the yogurt and season with freshly ground black pepper.

Heat a cast-iron skillet over high heat and lightly spray with the oil. Cook the tuna steaks for 2 minutes on each side, or until cooked, but still pink in the center.

Meanwhile, steam the vegetables for 2–3 minutes, or until just tender.

Top the tuna with the sauce. Serve with the vegetables and bread rolls.

HINT:
• Jalapeño chilies are smooth and thick-fleshed and are available both red and green. They are quite fiery, so you can use a less powerful variety of chili if you prefer.

THIS DELICIOUS MEAL IS QUICK AND
EASY TO MAKE AND PROVIDES USEFUL
AMOUNTS OF NUTRIENTS THAT MANY
PEOPLE DON'T EAT ENOUGH OF—
OMEGA-3 FATTY ACIDS, IRON, ZINC AND
OTHER MINERALS.

nutrition per serving: Energy 460 Cal
Fat 12.3 g
Saturated fat 4 g
Protein 51.1 g
Carbohydrate 32.1 g
Fiber 5.6 g
Cholesterol 61 mg

119

GREEN LENTIL AND VEGETABLE CURRY

IF YOU LIKE A LITTLE SPICE IN YOUR MEALS THIS ONE'S PERFECT. IT'S LOW GI, RICH IN FIBER AND ALSO CONTAINS A RANGE OF HEALTHY PLANT FOOD COMPOUNDS.

1 tsp olive or canola oil
1 large onion, chopped
2 garlic cloves, chopped
1–2 tbsp curry paste
1 tsp ground turmeric
1 cup green lentils, rinsed and drained
5 cups reduced-salt vegetable stock
1 large carrot, cut into ¾ in cubes
2 medium sweet potato, peeled and cut into ¾ in cubes
2 zucchini, cut into ¾ in slices

2 baby eggplants, cut into ½ in slices
basmati or wild rice, to serve (see Hint)
basil, to serve
cilantro leaves, to serve

PREP TIME: 20 MINUTES
COOKING TIME: 1 HOUR 5 MINUTES
SERVINGS: 4

Heat the oil in a saucepan over a medium heat. Add the onion and garlic and cook for 3 minutes, or until softened. Stir in the curry paste and turmeric and stir for 1 minute. Add the lentils and stock or water.

Bring to a boil, then reduce the heat. Cover and simmer for 30 minutes, then add the carrot and sweet potato. Simmer, covered, for 20 minutes, or until the lentils and vegetables are tender.

Add the zucchini and eggplant, cover and simmer for 10 minutes, or until the vegetables are cooked and most of the liquid has been absorbed. Remove the lid and simmer for a further few minutes if there is too much liquid. Serve hot with basmati rice or wild rice and top with basil and coriander leaves.

HINT:
• The rice will add a lot more carbohydrate, so if you have difficulty controlling your blood sugar level make sure that you have no more than 1 cup of cooked rice.

nutrition per serving: Energy 316 Cal; Fat 6.2 g; Saturated fat 0.8 g; Protein 16.9 g; Carbohydrate 43.2 g; Fiber 15.2 g; Cholesterol 0 mg

CILANTRO BEEF WITH NOODLES

MARINATE THE BEEF OVERNIGHT OR DURING THE DAY TO ALLOW THE FLAVORS TO DEVELOP IN THIS TASTY DISH. THE LIME JUICE AND CORIANDER GIVE A TANGY FLAVOR BOOST.

MARINADE
4 garlic cloves, finely chopped
1 tbsp finely chopped fresh ginger
1 large handful cilantro roots, stems and leaves, chopped
3 tsp olive or canola oil

about 1 lb lean beef rump steak
14 oz fresh rice noodles
olive or canola oil spray
1 red onion, thinly sliced

½ red pepper, thinly sliced
½ green pepper, thinly sliced
2 tbsp lime juice
2 tbsp reduced-sodium soy sauce
1 large handful cilantro leaves, extra

PREP TIME: 20 MINUTES + 2 HOURS MARINATING
COOKING TIME: 20 MINUTES
SERVINGS: 4

To make the marinade, combine the garlic, ginger, cilantro and 2 teaspoons of the oil in a large non-metallic bowl. Trim the beef, then cut into thin strips across the grain. Add to the marinade and toss to coat. Cover with plastic wrap and refrigerate for 2 hours, or overnight.

Put the rice noodles in a large heatproof bowl, cover with boiling water and soak for 8 minutes, or until softened. Separate gently and drain.

Heat a wok until very hot over high heat and spray with the oil. Add the meat in three batches and stir-fry for 2–3 minutes, or until the meat is just cooked. Remove all the meat from the wok and keep it warm. Reheat and respray the wok between batches.

Heat the remaining 1 teaspoon of oil in the wok. Add the onion and cook over medium heat for 3–4 minutes, or until slightly softened. Add the pepper and cook, tossing constantly, for 3–4 minutes, or until slightly softened.

Return all the meat to the wok along with the lime juice, soy sauce, 2 tablespoons of water and extra cilantro. Add the noodles. Toss well, then remove from the heat and season well with freshly ground black pepper.

nutrition per serving: Energy 409 Cal; Fat 10.4 g; Saturated fat 2.8 g; Protein 32.6 g; Carbohydrate 43.9 g; Fiber 2.2 g; Cholesterol 80 mg

121

THIS LOWER FAT, HEALTHIER VERSION OF
CHICKEN AND CHIPS IS RICH WITH EXOTIC
FLAVORS. THE DIFFERENT VEGETABLES GIVE
YOU A RANGE OF ANTIOXIDANTS AND
PHYTOCHEMICALS.

nutrition per serving: Energy 481 Cal
Fat 13.6 g
Saturated fat 3.7 g
Protein 41 g
Carbohydrate 44.4 g
Fiber 7.2 g
Cholesterol 155 mg

CAJUN CHICKEN WITH SALSA

4 sweet potatoes, peeled and cut into
   1¼ in chunks
olive or canola oil spray
4 skinless chicken thighs on the bone
4 skinless chicken drumsticks
3 tbsp Cajun seasoning
lime wedges, to serve

SALSA
3 cobs sweet corn
1 Lebanese (short) cucumber, cut into
   ¼ in dice

2 vine-ripened tomatoes, cut into ¼ in dice
1 small handful cilantro leaves, roughly
   chopped
2 tbsp lime juice
1 tsp fish sauce

PREP TIME: 25 MINUTES
COOKING TIME: 50 MINUTES
SERVINGS: 4

Preheat the oven to 350°F. Spray the sweet potatoes with the oil and season. Place in a roasting pan and roast in the oven for 40–45 minutes, or until golden and cooked through.

Put the chicken in a large bowl, add the Cajun seasoning mix and toss together well until the pieces are evenly coated. Place into a roasting pan and roast in the oven for 45 minutes, or until cooked through.

To make the salsa, cook the corn in a saucepan of boiling water for 8 minutes. Drain and refresh under cold water. Remove the kernels, using a sharp knife, and place in a bowl with the cucumber, tomato, coriander, lime juice and fish sauce. Mix together and season with pepper.

Serve the chicken pieces with the roasted sweet potato, the salsa and lime wedges.

SHRIMP JAMBALAYA

JAMBALAYA IS A VERSATILE CREOLE DISH THAT COMBINES COOKED RICE WITH A VARIETY OF VEGETABLES PLUS ANY KIND OF MEAT, POULTRY OR SEAFOOD. THIS SHRIMP-BASED VERSION IS LOW IN FAT AND PROVIDES GOOD AMOUNTS OF IODINE, SELENIUM AND ZINC.

about 2 lbs large shrimp, peeled and deveined, heads, shells and tails reserved
2 small onions, chopped
2 sticks celery, chopped
1 cup reduced-salt chicken stock
1 tbsp olive or canola oil
4½ oz low-fat bacon (we used 97% fat-free), thinly sliced
1 red pepper, chopped
15 oz canned chopped tomatoes

½ tsp cayenne pepper
½ tsp black pepper
¼ tsp dried thyme
¼ tsp dried oregano
2 cups basmati or doongara rice

PREP TIME: 25 MINUTES
COOKING TIME: 1 HOUR 10 MINUTES
SERVINGS: 4–6

Put the shrimp heads, shells and tails in a saucepan with half the onion, half the celery, the stock and 4 cups of water. Bring to a boil, then reduce the heat and simmer for 20 minutes. Strain through a fine sieve, reserving the shrimp stock.

Heat the oil in a large, heavy-based saucepan and cook the bacon for 3 minutes, or until lightly browned. Remove from the saucepan with a slotted spoon and set aside.

Add the remaining onion, the remaining celery and the pepper to the saucepan and cook, stirring occasionally, for 5 minutes. Add the tomato, cayenne pepper, black pepper and dried herbs and bring to a boil. Reduce the heat and simmer, covered, for 10 minutes.

Return the bacon to the pan and add the rice and shrimp stock. Bring back to a boil, reduce the heat and simmer, covered, for 25 minutes, or until most of the liquid has been absorbed and the rice is tender.

Add the shrimp to the saucepan and stir through gently. Cover and cook for a further 5 minutes, or until the shrimp are pink and cooked through. Serve immediately.

nutrition per serving (6): Energy 400 Cal; Fat 4.8 g; Saturated fat 0.7 g; Protein 29.5 g; Carbohydrate 58.3 g; Fiber 2.3 g; Cholesterol 144 mg

CHILI CON CARNE

THIS SPICY CLASSIC PROVIDES A SUSTAINING LOW-GI MEAL WITH SIGNIFICANT AMOUNTS OF VITAMIN C, FOLATE, BETACAROTENE, B-GROUP VITAMINS, IRON AND ZINC.

2 tsp olive or canola oil
1 large onion, chopped
1 garlic clove, crushed
1 tsp cayenne pepper
2 tsp paprika
1 tsp dried oregano
2 tsp ground cumin
1½ to 2 lbs extra lean ground beef
1½ cups reduced-salt
  beef stock
15 oz canned diced tomatoes

½ cup no-added-salt tomato paste
10½ oz canned kidney beans, drained and
  rinsed
fresh flat-leaf (Italian) parsley sprigs,
  to garnish
basmati or doongar rice, to serve
  (see Hint)

PREP TIME: 15 MINUTES
COOKING TIME: 1 HOUR 10 MINUTES
SERVINGS: 6

Heat the oil in a saucepan over low heat. Add the onion and cook for 4–5 minutes, or until soft. Stir in the garlic, cayenne pepper, paprika, oregano and cumin. Increase the heat to medium, add the beef and cook for 5–8 minutes, or until just browned.

Reduce the heat to low and add the stock, tomato and tomato paste. Cook for 40 minutes, stirring frequently.

Stir in the kidney beans and simmer for 10 minutes. Serve the chili con carne on its own in small bowls or over steamed basmati or doongara rice. Garnish with a sprig of parsley.

HINT:
• The rice will add more carbohydrate, so choose a small serve.

nutrition per serving: Energy 276 Cal; Fat 10.4 g; Saturated fat 3.9 g; Protein 30.3 g; Carbohydrate 11.7 g; Fiber 4.7 g; Cholesterol 65 mg

REDUCED-FAT LASAGNA

2 tsp olive or canola oil
1 large onion, chopped
2 carrots, finely chopped
2 celery stalks, finely chopped
2 zucchini, finely chopped
2 garlic cloves, crushed
about 1 lb lean ground beef
28 oz canned chopped tomatoes
½ cup reduced-salt beef stock
2 tbsp no-added-salt tomato paste
2 tsp dried oregano

16 oz no-boil lasagna sheets
mixed-leaf salad with balsamic vinegar,
    to serve

CHEESE SAUCE
3 cups skim milk
⅓ cup cornstarch
3½ oz reduced-fat cheddar cheese

PREP TIME: 40 MINUTES
COOKING TIME: 1 HOUR 35 MINUTES
SERVINGS: 8

Heat the oil in a large non-stick saucepan over medium heat. Add the onion and cook for 5 minutes, or until soft. Add the carrot, celery and zucchini and cook, stirring constantly, for 5 minutes, or until soft. Add the garlic and cook for 1 minute. Increase the heat to high, add the beef and cook, stirring, until well browned. Break up any lumps with a wooden spoon. Add the tomato, stock, tomato paste and oregano to the pan and stir well. Bring to a boil, then reduce the heat and simmer gently, partially covered, for 20 minutes, stirring occasionally to prevent the mixture sticking to the pan.

Preheat the oven to 350°F. Spread a little of the meat sauce into the base of a 9 x 13 in ovenproof dish. Arrange a layer of lasagna sheets in the dish, breaking some of the sheets, if necessary, to fit in neatly. Spread half the meat sauce over the top to cover evenly. Cover with another layer of lasagna sheets, a layer of meat sauce, then a final layer of lasagna sheets.

To make the cheese sauce, blend a little of the milk with the cornstarch, to form a smooth paste, in a small saucepan. Gradually blend in the remaining milk and stir constantly over low heat until the mixture boils and thickens. Remove from the heat and stir in the cheese until melted.

Spread the sauce evenly over the top of the lasagna. Bake for 1 hour, checking after 25 minutes. If the top is browning too quickly, cover loosely with non-stick baking paper or foil sprayed with oil. Take care when removing the paper or foil that the topping does not lift off. Serve with the mixed-leaf salad.

A PERENNIAL FAVORITE, THIS VERSION
HAS ALL THE FLAVOR BUT LESS FAT
THAN TRADITIONAL LASAGNA—BUT YOU
STILL NEED TO LIMIT YOURSELF TO ONE
PORTION.

nutrition per serving: Energy 333 Cal
Fat 9 g
Saturated fat 3.8 g
Protein 26.1 g
Carbohydrate 35.3 g
Fiber 5 g
Cholesterol 43 mg

SPAGHETTI BOLOGNESE

THIS IS A LOW-GI DISH THE WHOLE FAMILY WILL ENJOY. MEATY SAUCE GOES WELL WITH MOST TYPES OF PASTA, SO YOU CAN SWAP THE SPAGHETTI WITH OTHER TYPES OF PASTA FOR A NEW TWIST.

olive or canola oil spray
2 onions, finely chopped
2 garlic cloves, finely chopped
2 carrots, finely chopped
2 celery stalks, finely chopped
about 1 lb lean ground beef
4 to 5 tomatoes, chopped
½ cup red wine (see Hints)
12 oz spaghetti

3 tbsp finely chopped flat-leaf (Italian) parsley
mixed-leaf salad with balsamic vinegar, to serve

PREP TIME: 20 MINUTES
COOKING TIME: 1 HOUR 20 MINUTES
SERVINGS: 6

Heat a large saucepan over medium heat. Spray with the oil, then add the onion, garlic, carrot and celery. Stir for 5 minutes, or until the vegetables have softened. Add 1 tablespoon water, if necessary, to prevent sticking.

Increase the heat to high, add the beef and cook for 5 minutes, or until browned. Stir constantly to prevent the meat sticking. Add the tomatoes, wine and 1 cup water. Bring to a boil, reduce the heat and simmer, uncovered, for about 1 hour, until the sauce has thickened.

Meanwhile, cook the spaghetti in a large saucepan of boiling water for 10 minutes, or until *al dente*. Drain. Stir the parsley through the sauce, season with salt and freshly ground black pepper and serve over the pasta. Serve with the mixed-leaf salad.

HINTS:
• This dish tastes even better the next day and can be kept in the fridge for up to 2 days or frozen for up to 1 month.
• If you'd prefer not to use wine, the same amount of liquid can be replaced with reduced-salt beef stock.
• Choose wholemeal pasta if you're watching your weight to make this meal more filling.

nutrition per serving: Energy 357 Cal; Fat 5.9 g; Saturated fat 2.1 g; Protein 22.6 g; Carbohydrate 46.3 g; Fiber 5.5 g; Cholesterol 34 mg

MOUSSAKA

THIS LOW-FAT VERSION OF A GREEK FAVORITE MAKES A NOURISHING, LOW-GI MEAL, PROVIDING GOOD AMOUNTS OF IRON, ZINC, CALCIUM, PHOSPHORUS, PROTEIN AND VARIOUS ANTIOXIDANTS.

2 to 3 eggplants
olive or canola oil spray
2 onions, finely chopped
3 large garlic cloves, crushed
$\frac{1}{2}$ tsp ground allspice
1 tsp ground cinnamon
about 1 lb lean ground lamb
2 tbsp no-added-salt tomato paste
$\frac{1}{2}$ cup reduced-salt vegetable or beef stock
28 oz canned tomatoes
3 tbsp chopped flat-leaf (Italian) parsley
$3\frac{1}{4}$ oz low-fat cheddar cheese, grated

1 tbsp reduced-fat olive oil or canola oil margarine
$\frac{1}{3}$ cup all-purpose flour
$1\frac{1}{2}$ cups skim milk
$\frac{2}{3}$ cup low-fat ricotta cheese
pinch ground nutmeg

PREP TIME: 30 MINUTES

COOKING TIME: 1 HOUR 30 MINUTES

SERVINGS: 6

Preheat the oven to 350°F. Cut the eggplant into $\frac{1}{4}$ in thick slices. Spray the eggplant with the oil and broil under a preheated broiler for 4 minutes on each side, or until golden.

Heat a non-stick saucepan and lightly spray with oil. Cook the onions for 3–4 minutes, or until softened. Add the garlic, allspice and cinnamon and cook for 1 minute. Add the lamb and cook for 3–4 minutes, or until cooked. Add the tomato paste, stock and tomatoes. Bring to a boil, then reduce the heat and simmer for 30–35 minutes, stirring occasionally, or until most of the liquid has evaporated. Stir in the parsley and season.

To make the white sauce, melt the margarine in a saucepan over medium heat. Stir in the flour and cook for 1 minute. Remove from the heat and gradually stir in the milk. Return to the heat and stir constantly until the sauce boils and thickens. Reduce the heat and simmer for 2 minutes. Stir through the ricotta and nutmeg until smooth and season with freshly ground black pepper.

Spoon half the meat sauce into a 12-cup ovenproof dish. Cover with half of the eggplant. Spoon over the remaining meat sauce and cover with the remaining eggplant. Spread over the sauce and sprinkle with the cheese. Bake for 30 minutes, or until golden.

nutrition per serving: Energy 337 Cal; Fat 12.5 g; Saturated fat 4.5 g; Protein 31.4 g; Carbohydrate 21.1 g; Fiber 7.3; Cholesterol 66 mg

THIS IS A GOOD WEEKDAY RECIPE BECAUSE IT DOESN'T TAKE LONG TO PREPARE. IT'S LOW GI AND A GOOD SOURCE OF FIBER, FOLATE, BETACAROTENE AND LYCOPENE.

nutrition per serving: Energy 505 Cal

Fat 4.4 g

Saturated fat 0.6 g

Protein 16.6 g

Carbohydrate 94.5 g

Fiber 7.2 g

Cholesterol 2 mg

PASTA PUTTANESCA

2 tsp olive or canola oil

3 garlic cloves, crushed

2 tbsp chopped flat-leaf (Italian) parsley

$\frac{1}{4}$–$\frac{1}{2}$ tsp chili flakes or powder

28 oz canned chopped tomatoes

16 oz spaghetti

1 tbsp capers

3 anchovy fillets in brine, drained and thinly sliced

$\frac{1}{4}$ cup black olives in brine, drained, pitted and chopped

mixed-leaf salad with balsamic vinegar, to serve

PREP TIME: 20 MINUTES

COOKING TIME: 25 MINUTES

SERVINGS: 4

Heat the oil in a large heavy-based frying pan. Add the garlic, parsley and chili flakes and stir constantly for about 1 minute over medium heat. Add the tomato to the pan and bring to a boil. Reduce the heat and simmer, covered, for 10 minutes.

Meanwhile, cook the pasta in a large saucepan of boiling water for 10 minutes, or until *al dente*. Drain and return to the pan.

Add the capers, anchovies and olives to the tomato mixture and stir for a further 5 minutes. Season with freshly ground black pepper. Add the sauce to the pasta and toss gently. Serve with the mixed-leaf salad.

HINTS:
- You can substitute the anchovies with a small–medium tin of tuna if you don't like anchovies.
- Less active people need to make sure that they don't overdo the pasta—so eat less pasta and more sauce and salad for a more filling meal.

PENNE WITH SEARED TUNA AND ZUCCHINI

THIS LOW-FAT, MEDITERRANEAN-STYLE DISH WITH A HINT OF ZESTY LEMON PROVIDES PLENTY OF PROTEIN, OMEGA-3 FATTY ACIDS, NIACIN, POTASSIUM, FOLATE, AND SOME IRON AND ZINC.

14 oz penne pasta
olive or canola oil spray
about 1 lb tuna steaks
1 large red onion, cut into thin wedges
2 zucchini, sliced into 2¾ in long thin strips
1 garlic clove, chopped
6 small gherkins, rinsed and chopped

1 large handful flat-leaf (Italian) parsley, chopped
zest and juice from 1 large lemon
mixed-leaf salad with balsamic vinegar, to serve

PREP TIME: 15 MINUTES
COOKING TIME: 20 MINUTES
SERVINGS: 4

Cook the pasta in a large saucepan of boiling salted water for 10 minutes, or until *al dente*. Drain, reserving 1 cup of the pasta water. Return the pasta to the saucepan.

Meanwhile, pat the fish dry with paper towels. Lightly spray a large, non-stick frying pan with the oil. Heat the oil, add the fish and cook for 2–3 minutes on each side, or until browned on the outside and still pink in the center. Remove the fish from the pan. Set aside for a few minutes, then cut into ¾ in cubes.

Spray the frying pan with more oil and heat the pan. Add the onion, zucchini and garlic and cook for 2–3 minutes, or until softened. Stir in the gherkins, parsley, lemon zest and juice. Toss into the hot pasta together with the fish and enough of the reserved pasta water to moisten. Season with freshly ground black pepper. Serve with the mixed-leaf salad.

HINT:
• If you generally have trouble keeping your blood sugar level under control, make sure you have a smaller serve of pasta. If you feel like seconds, fill up on salad.

nutrition per serving: Energy 600 Cal; Fat 9.5 g; Saturated fat 3.2 g; Protein 44.2 g; Carbohydrate 79.4 g; Fiber 6.1 g; Cholesterol 45 mg

LENTIL AND RICOTTA LASAGNA

THIS DISH IS LOWER IN FAT THAN REGULAR LASAGNA AND CONTAINS MORE FIBER. IT IS ALSO LOW IN SATURATED FAT.

$\frac{1}{2}$ cup red lentils

1 large onion

1 small red pepper

2 zucchini

1 celery stalk

2 tsp olive or canola oil

2–3 garlic cloves, crushed

28 oz canned chopped tomatoes

2 tbsp no-added-salt tomato paste

1 tsp dried oregano

$\frac{1}{3}$ cup cornstarch

3 cups skim milk

$\frac{1}{4}$ onion

$\frac{1}{2}$ tsp ground nutmeg

$1\frac{1}{3}$ cups low-fat ricotta cheese

12 dried or fresh lasagna sheets

$\frac{1}{2}$ cup grated reduced-fat cheddar cheese

PREP TIME: 30 MINUTES + 30 MINUTES
    SOAKING

COOKING TIME: 1 HOUR 50 MINUTES

SERVINGS: 6

Pour the lentils into a bowl, cover with boiling water and leave to soak for 30 minutes. Drain. Chop the onion and pepper, then slice the zucchini and celery. Heat the oil in a saucepan, add the garlic and onion and cook for 2 minutes. Add the pepper, zucchini and celery and cook for 2–3 minutes, or until softened. Add the lentils, tomatoes, tomato paste, oregano and $1\frac{1}{2}$ cups water. Bring to a boil, then reduce the heat and simmer for 30 minutes, or until the lentils are tender. Preheat the oven to 350°F.

Blend the cornstarch with 2 tablespoons of the milk in a saucepan until smooth. Pour the remaining milk into the pan. Add the onion and stir over low heat until the mixture boils and thickens. Add the nutmeg and season with freshly ground black pepper, then cook over low heat for 5 minutes. Remove the onion.

Beat the ricotta with $\frac{1}{2}$ cup of the white sauce. Spread one-third of the lentil mixture over the base of a 12-cup ovenproof dish. Cover with a layer of lasagna sheets. Spread another third of the lentil mixture over the pasta, then spread the ricotta over the top. Follow with another layer of lasagna, then the remaining lentils.

Pour the white sauce over the top. Sprinkle with the grated cheese. Bake for 1 hour, covering with lightly oiled foil if the top starts to brown too much. Stand for 5 minutes before cutting.

nutrition per serving: Energy 397 Cal; Fat 7.9 g; Saturated fat 2.9 g; Protein 23.7 g; Carbohydrate 55.1 g; Fiber 6.8 g; Cholesterol 10 mg

COQ AU VIN

2 tsp olive or canola oil

4½ oz low-fat bacon (we used
   97% fat-free), roughly chopped

about 3½ lbs skinless chicken pieces,
   trimmed

12 oz baby onions

2 tbsp all-purpose flour

3 cups reduced-salt beef stock

9 oz field mushrooms, sliced

1 tbsp thyme, to garnish

6 wholegrain bread rolls

PREP TIME: 15 MINUTES

COOKING TIME: 1 HOUR 50 MINUTES

SERVINGS: 6

Preheat the oven to 350°F. Heat the oil in a large flameproof casserole dish. Add the bacon and cook until golden, then remove. Add the chicken in batches and cook for 4–5 minutes, or until browned. Remove from the dish. Add the onions and cook for 2–3 minutes, or until browned, then remove from the dish.

Add the flour to the dish and stir well, then remove from the heat and slowly stir in the stock. Return to the heat, bring to a boil and return the bacon and chicken to the pan. Cover and cook in the oven for 1 hour. Return the onions to the pan and add the mushrooms. Cook for a further 30 minutes. Season to taste with freshly ground black pepper, then garnish with the thyme.

Meanwhile, put the bread rolls in the oven for a few minutes, or until warmed through. Serve with the casserole.

HINT:
• For extra filling power and antioxidants, serve with a medley of steamed vegetables, such as broccoli, cauliflower, squash, carrots and zucchini.

THIS RECIPE CONTAINS LESS FAT THAN
THE TRADITIONAL FRENCH VERSION OF
COQ AU VIN, BUT STILL HAS ALL THE
FLAVOR. IT'S GREAT AS LEFTOVERS.

nutrition per serving: Energy 515 Cal

Fat 19.4 g

Saturated fat 5.6 g

Protein 49.2 g

Carbohydrate 34 g

Fiber 5.2 g

Cholesterol 150 mg

OSSO BUCCO WITH GREMOLATA

A GREAT WINTER WARMER, OSSO BUCCO CAN BE SERVED WITH PASTA OR GRAINY BREAD FOR A NOURISHING LOW-GI MEAL.

GREMOLATA
1 tbsp finely shredded lemon zest
1–2 garlic cloves, finely chopped
3 tbsp finely chopped flat-leaf (Italian) parsley

all-purpose flour, for dusting
4 lean veal shank pieces, 2 in thick
2 tsp olive or canola oil
2 large onions, sliced
6 roma (plum) tomatoes, finely chopped
2 tbsp no-added-salt tomato paste

1½ cups white wine
1 tbsp cornstarch
2–3 garlic cloves, crushed
¼ cup flat-leaf (Italian) parsley, finely chopped
14 oz penne
mixed-leaf salad with balsamic vinegar, to serve

PREP TIME: 40 MINUTES
COOKING TIME: 2½ HOURS
SERVINGS: 4

To make the gremolata, mix together the lemon zest, garlic and parsley and set aside.

Season the flour with a little salt and freshly ground black pepper. Toss the veal pieces in the flour, shaking off any excess. Heat half the oil in a large, heavy-based frying pan. When the oil is hot, brown the veal on both sides. Remove and set aside.

Heat the remaining oil in the pan and cook the onion for 2–3 minutes, or until soft but not brown. Add the meat in a single layer so that it fits snugly in the pan. Season with freshly ground black pepper.

Mix together the tomatoes, tomato paste and wine and pour the mixture over the meat. Bring to a boil, then reduce the heat, cover and simmer for 1½ hours.

Remove 1 cup of the cooking liquid and set aside to cool slightly. Put the cornstarch in a small bowl and whisk in the reserved liquid, then stir in the garlic and chopped parsley and add the mixture to the pan. Simmer, uncovered, for about 30 minutes, or until the meat is very tender and the sauce has thickened. Sprinkle with the gremolata just before serving.

Meanwhile, cook the pasta in a large saucepan of boiling water for 10 minutes, or until *al dente*. Drain well. Serve with the mixed-leaf salad.

nutrition per serving: Energy 588 Cal; Fat 6.5 g; Saturated fat 1.3 g; Protein 33.4 g; Carbohydrate 77.1 g; Fiber 7.5 g; Cholesterol 75 mg

CHILI BEANS WITH POLENTA

SUITABLE FOR VEGETARIANS WHO EAT DAIRY PRODUCTS, THIS DELIGHTFULLY SPICY DISH IS RICH IN FIBER AND PROVIDES COMPLETE PROTEIN PLUS GOOD AMOUNTS OF FIBER AND ANTIOXIDANTS.

14½ oz canned creamed corn
½ cup instant polenta (see Hint)
10½ oz canned corn kernels, drained
⅓ cup low-fat, vintage cheddar cheese, grated
1 tbsp chopped cilantro leaves
1 tbsp olive oil
1 red onion, sliced
2 garlic cloves, crushed
1 tsp chili powder
1 tsp paprika
1 tbsp ground cumin
1 tsp ground coriander

14 oz canned kidney beans, rinsed and drained
14 oz canned borlotti beans, rinsed and drained
28 oz canned tomatoes
2 tbsp no-added-salt tomato paste
2 tbsp chopped cilantro leaves

PREP TIME: 15 MINUTES
COOKING TIME: 35 MINUTES
SERVINGS: 6

Line an 8 in round cake pan with plastic wrap. Place the creamed corn and stock in a saucepan and bring to a boil. Stir in the polenta and corn kernels, and cook over medium heat until it comes away from the sides. Stir in the cheese and cilantro, cool for 5 minutes, then spoon into the tin and level the surface. Cool.

Heat the oil in a large saucepan, add the onion, garlic and spices and cook until soft. Stir in the beans, tomato and tomato paste. Simmer for 20 minutes. Stir in the cilantro.

Lift the polenta from the pan with the aid of the plastic wrap, cut into wedges and serve with the chili beans and a salad on the side.

HINT:
• The coarser the polenta, the lower the GI (using a thicker polenta rather than very fine instant polenta is recommeneded).

nutrition per serving: Energy 327 Cal; Fat 5.9 g; Saturated fat 1.1 g; Protein 13.8 g; Carbohydrate 50 g; Fiber 11.2 g; Cholesterol 7 mg

THIS DISH IS HEALTHIER THAN FISH
AND CHIPS WITH MUCH LESS FAT AND
MORE NUTRIENTS. IT COMBINES THE
FILLING POWERS OF FISH AND LENTILS
TO GIVE YOU A VERY SATISFYING MEAL.

nutrition per serving: Energy 338 Cal
Fat 10.4 g
Saturated fat 0.8 g
Protein 36.6 g
Carbohydrate 21.1 g
Fiber 6 g
Cholesterol 49 mg

CRISPY FISH AND LENTILS

⅓ cup all-purpose flour

about 1½ lbs boneless white
   fish fillets

2 tbsp olive or canola oil

4 spring onions (scallions), diagonally
   sliced

2 garlic cloves, crushed

28 oz canned brown lentils, drained

9 oz green beans, trimmed

PREP TIME: 10 MINUTES

COOKING TIME: 15 MINUTES

SERVINGS: 4

Coat the fish fillets in the flour, shaking off any excess. Heat 1 tablespoon of the oil in a large, non-stick frying pan over medium–high heat. Add the fish and cook for 3–4 minutes on each side, or until cooked through and lightly browned—depending on the size of your frying pan you may need to cook the fish in batches.

Meanwhile, heat the remaining oil in a large saucepan. Cook the spring onions and garlic for 2 minutes, or until softened. Add the lentils. Toss for a few minutes, or until the lentils are heated through.

Steam or microwave the beans for a few minutes, or until just tender.

Serve the fish with the warm lentils and green beans.

HINT:
• You could serve this dish with extra vegetables, such as mushrooms, broccoli, cauliflower or spinach if you want a more filling meal.

ROAST CHICKEN WITH VEGETABLES

INSTEAD OF THE TRADITIONAL STAPLE OF ROAST MEAT AND THREE VEGGIES, TRY THIS DISH OF CHICKEN WITH FIVE DIFFERENT TYPES OF VEGETABLES. IT HAS MORE NUTRIENTS AND COLOR.

1 x 3 lb chicken
1 lemon, halved
6 garlic cloves, unpeeled
6 sprigs thyme
2 medium sweet potatoes, cut into 2 in pieces
2 large carrots, peeled and cut into 2 in pieces
olive or canola oil spray
2 tbsp all-purpose flour
1 tbsp Dijon mustard

1½ cups salt-reduced chicken stock
4 corn cobs, trimmed
large bunch (about 14 oz) broccoli, cut into florets
2 zucchini, cut into 1¼ in pieces

PREP TIME: 30 MINUTES
COOKING TIME: 1 HOUR 10 MINUTES
SERVINGS: 4–6

Preheat the oven to 400°F. Season the chicken and place the lemon in the cavity. Bend the wings back and tuck behind the body of the chicken. Tie the drumsticks together using string or skewers. Place the chicken in a large roasting pan and arrange the garlic, thyme, sweet potato and carrot around it. Spray the chicken and vegetables with the oil, and bake for 1 hour, or until the chicken is tender and the juices run clear. Turn the vegetables after 30 minutes.

Transfer the chicken and vegetables, except the garlic, to separate plates, cover and keep warm. In a large saucepan of boiling water, cook the corn for 8 minutes. Steam the broccoli and zucchini until just tender.

Meanwhile, pour off any excess fat from the roasting pan. Peel the garlic and mash with a fork in the tin. Heat the tin on the stove top, add the flour and cook over medium heat, stirring, until golden. Remove from the heat and stir in the mustard and stock. Return to the heat and stir until the gravy boils and thickens. Carve the chicken and serve skinless portions of meat with the gravy, roast vegetables, corn, broccoli and zucchini.

HINTS:
• Microwave the corn, beans and zucchini if you prefer.
• Make sure you serve the chicken without the skin—that's where most of the fat is.

nutrition per serving: Energy 587 Cal; Fat 18 g; Saturated fat 4.7 g; Protein 61.2 g; Carbohydrate 38.8 g; Fiber 11.2 g; Cholesterol 188 mg

PEPPER BEEF ON CANNELLINI BEAN MASH

THIS STEAK RECIPE IS LOW IN FAT BUT RICH IN FLAVOR AND IS A GOOD SOURCE OF FIBER, PROTEIN, IRON AND ZINC.

6 garlic cloves, unpeeled

2 tbsp whole black peppercorns

¼ tsp or less sea salt

5½ oz lean beef fillet steaks, trimmed

olive or canola oil spray

large bunch (about 1 lb) broccoli, cut into florets

4 tbsp reduced-salt vegetable stock

28 oz canned cannellini beans, rinsed and drained

2 tbsp chopped flat-leaf (Italian) parsley

10½ oz baby spinach leaves, trimmed

PREP TIME: 15 MINUTES
COOKING TIME: 40 MINUTES
SERVINGS: 4

Preheat the oven to 350°F. Roast the garlic on a tray for 20 minutes, or until softened.

Place the peppercorns in a spice grinder (or use a mortar and pestle) with the sea salt, and roughly crush. Put on a plate, then roll the steaks in the mix until they are well coated.

Over medium heat, heat a chargrill pan, spray with the oil, then add the steaks. Cook for 5 minutes on each side for a medium–rare steak. Remove from the pan and rest, covered, for 2 minutes. Steam or microwave the broccoli for 3 minutes, or until just tender.

Squeeze the garlic from the skin and discard the skin. In a saucepan, bring the vegetable stock to a boil. Add the cannellini beans and garlic and roughly crush together, using a fork, until mashed but still quite chunky. When heated stir through the parsley.

Place the spinach in a saucepan with 2 teaspoons water, cover and place over low–medium heat and cook for 1 minute, or until the leaves are just beginning to wilt. Remove from the heat, stir and season well with freshly ground black pepper.

To serve, divide the bean mash and broccoli between 4 serving plates, top the mash with the spinach and sit the fillet on top. Drizzle with any of the juices which may have come from the resting steaks.

nutrition per serving: Energy 402 Cal; Fat 9.8 g; Saturated fat 3.6 g; Protein 51.7 g; Carbohydrate 19.5 g; Fiber 16.9 g; Cholesterol 109 mg

SLOW-COOKED LAMB SHANKS WITH BARLEY

2 tsp olive or canola oil
4 lean lamb shanks
2 red onions, sliced
10 garlic cloves, peeled
15 oz canned chopped tomatoes
$\frac{1}{2}$ cup reduced-salt vegetable stock or dry
   white wine
1 bay leaf
1 tsp grated lemon zest

1 large red pepper, chopped
$1\frac{1}{2}$ cups pearl barley
3 tbsp chopped flat-leaf (Italian) parsley
mixed-leaf salad with balsamic vinegar,
   to serve

PREP TIME: 20 MINUTES
COOKING TIME: 3¼ HOURS
SERVINGS: 4

Preheat the oven to 325°F. Heat the oil in a large flameproof casserole dish, add the shanks in batches and cook over high heat until browned on all sides. Remove the lamb to a side plate.

Add the onion and garlic to the dish and cook until softened. Return all the lamb to the casserole dish. Add the tomato, wine, bay leaf, lemon zest, pepper and $\frac{1}{2}$ cup water and bring to a boil. Cover the dish and cook in the oven for 2–2$\frac{1}{2}$ hours, or until the meat is tender and falling off the bone and the sauce has thickened.

Meanwhile, wash the barley, then drain well. Put it in a large saucepan with 5 cups water. Bring to a boil, then simmer for 30 minutes, or until soft. Drain.

Season the shanks with freshly ground black pepper to taste. Sprinkle the parsley over the top before serving. Serve with the barley and the salad.

HINT:
• Barley is a good source of soluble fiber and a very low-GI food—great for people with diabetes. It is very filling, so some people might find it difficult to eat at first.

THIS IS A PERFECT COUNTRY-STYLE
MEAL FOR COLD WINTER WEEKENDS.
THE LOW-GI, FIBER-RICH BARLEY WILL
KEEP YOU FULL FOR HOURS.

nutrition per serving: Energy 598 Cal
Fat 17.9 g
Saturated fat 6.6 g
Protein 39.5 g
Carbohydrate 57.8 g
Fiber 13 g
Cholesterol 95 mg

PORK AND BEAN CHILI

THIS DISH IS AN EASY WAY TO INCLUDE LEGUMES IN YOUR DIET.

olive or canola oil spray

about 1½ lbs lean pork fillet

1 small red onion, finely chopped

3 garlic cloves, finely chopped

1½ tsp ground cumin

1 tsp ground oregano

1–1½ tsp dried chili powder

2 tsp sweet paprika

1 tbsp red wine vinegar

28 oz canned kidney beans, drained and rinsed

15 oz canned Italian tomatoes

1½ cups reduced-salt beef stock

1 tbsp no-added-salt tomato paste

1 dried bay leaf

CORIANDER RICE

1¼ cups basmati or doongara rice

2–3 tbsp chopped cilantro leaves

PREP TIME: 15 MINUTES +10 MINUTES
   STANDING

COOKING TIME: 2 HOURS

SERVINGS: 4

Heat a large, non-stick saucepan over high heat. Cut the pork into 1 in cubes. Spray with the oil, then brown the pork in 2 batches for 2–3 minutes, or until evenly browned. Remove the pork. Reduce the heat to medium, spray the pan with the oil, then add the onion and cook for 4–5 minutes, or until soft. Stir in the garlic, cumin, oregano, chili and paprika. Add the vinegar and stir for 30 seconds, or until it evaporates.

Return the pork and any juices to the pan, then add the kidney beans, tomatoes and juice, stock, tomato paste and bay leaf. Stir to combine thoroughly and allow the mixture to come to a boil. Reduce the heat to very low and cook, covered, for 1 hour, stirring frequently. Remove the lid from the pan and continue to cook, uncovered, for a further 30 minutes, or until the meat is tender and the sauce has reduced and thickened.

Rinse the rice and put it in a saucepan. Add 2 cups water and bring to a boil. Cover, reduce the heat to low and cook for 10 minutes. Remove from the heat and leave to stand, covered, for 10 minutes.

Season the pork and bean chili with freshly ground black pepper. Stir the cilantro through the rice. Place the rice into 4 serving bowls, top with the pork and bean chili. Garnish with 2 tablespoons chopped flat-leaf (Italian) parsley, 1 tablespoon chopped cilantro and 2 teaspoons extra-light sour cream or low-fat yogurt per serving, if you like.

nutrition per serving: Energy 580 Cal; Fat 6.1 g; Saturated fat 1.6 g; Protein 48.8 g; Carbohydrate 75.1 g; Fiber 11.9 g; Cholesterol 144 mg

VEAL CUTLETS IN CHILI TOMATO SAUCE

SERVED WITH A SPICY TOMATO SAUCE, THIS LOW-GI VEAL DISH IS A PERFECT CHOICE FOR WINTER
NIGHTS. IT'S A GOOD SOURCE OF PROTEIN, B VITAMINS, FOLATE, POTASSIUM, IRON AND ZINC.

5 slices wholegrain bread
3 tbsp flat-leaf (Italian) parsley
3 garlic cloves
4 thick veal cutlets, trimmed
3 tbsp skim milk
2 tsp olive or canola oil
1 onion, finely chopped
1 tbsp capers, drained
1 tsp canned green peppercorns, chopped
1 tsp chopped red chili

2 tbsp balsamic vinegar
1 tsp brown sugar
2 tbsp no-added-salt tomato paste
15 oz canned chopped tomatoes

PREP TIME: 35 MINUTES
COOKING TIME: 35 MINUTES
SERVINGS: 4

Preheat the oven to 350°F. Place a rack in a small baking dish. Chop the bread, parsley and garlic in a food processor to make fine breadcrumbs.

Season the cutlets on both sides with a little salt and freshly ground black pepper. Pour the milk into a bowl and put the breadcrumbs on a plate. Dip the veal in the milk, then coat in the crumbs, pressing the crumbs on. Transfer to the rack and bake for 20 minutes.

Meanwhile, heat the oil in a small pan over medium heat. Add the onion, capers, peppercorns and chili, cover and cook for 8 minutes. Stir in the vinegar, sugar and tomato paste, and stir until boiling. Stir in the tomato, reduce the heat and simmer for 15 minutes, then season with pepper.

Remove the cutlets from the rack and wipe the dish. Place about three-quarters of the tomato sauce in the base and put the cutlets on top. Spoon the remaining sauce over the cutlets and return to the oven. Reduce the oven to 300°F, then bake for another 10 minutes, or until heated through. Sprinkle with extra chopped parsley.

nutrition per serving: Energy 314 Cal; Fat 6.9 g; Saturated fat 1.4 g; Protein 33.2 g; Carbohydrate 26.4 g; Fiber 4.9 g; Cholesterol 103 mg

THIS DISH IS A FRENCH CLASSIC—A
HEARTY STEW THAT IS BOTH FLAVORFUL
AND SATISFYING, AND MAKES DELICIOUS
LEFTOVERS.

nutrition per serving: Energy 524 Cal

Fat 9.7 g

Saturated fat 3.6 g

Protein 48.8 g

Carbohydrate 51.1 g

Fiber 3.4 g

Cholesterol 110 mg

BEEF BOURGUIGNON

about 2 lbs lean topside or round steak
all-purpose flour, for dusting
2 to 3 slices low-fat bacon (we used 97%
   fat-free)
2 tsp olive or canola oil
12 baby onions
1 cup red wine (see Hints)
2 cups reduced-salt beef stock
1 tsp dried thyme
7 oz button mushrooms

2 bay leaves
14 oz fettucine
mixed-leaf salad with balsamic vinegar,
   to serve

PREP TIME: 20 MINUTES
COOKING TIME: 2 HOURS
SERVINGS: 6

Trim the steak and cut into ¾ in cubes. Season the flour with a little salt and freshly ground black pepper. Lightly toss the steak in the flour, shaking off the excess.

Cut the bacon into ¾ in squares. Heat the oil in a large heavy-based saucepan and briefly cook the bacon over medium heat. Remove the bacon from the pan, then add the meat and brown well in batches. Remove and set aside. Add the onions to the pan and cook until golden.

Return the bacon and meat to the pan with the remaining ingredients (except the pasta and salad). Bring to a boil, reduce the heat and simmer, covered, for 1½ hours, or until the meat is very tender, stirring occasionally. Remove the bay leaves to serve.

Meanwhile, cook the pasta in a large saucepan of boiling water for 10 minutes, or until *al dente*. Drain well. Serve with the beef. Serve with the mixed-leaf salad.

HINTS:
• If you'd prefer not to use wine, the same amount of liquid can be replaced with extra reduced-salt beef stock.
• Great as leftovers, this dish will keep refrigerated in an airtight container for up to 3 days.

CHICKEN CHASSEUR

THIS NOURISHING STEW IS PERFECT IN COOL WEATHER. MAKE IT ON THE WEEKEND WHEN YOU HAVE PLENTY OF TIME TO ENJOY THE SUCCULENT AROMAS WHILE IT'S COOKING.

2 tsp olive or canola oil
about 2 lbs skinless chicken thigh fillets, trimmed
1 garlic clove, crushed
1 large onion, sliced
3½ oz button mushrooms, sliced
1 tsp thyme
15 oz canned tomatoes
3 tbsp reduced-salt chicken stock

3 tbsp white wine (optional)
1 tbsp no-added-salt tomato paste
14 oz penne

PREP TIME: 20 MINUTES

COOKING TIME: 1 HOUR 30 MINUTES

SERVINGS: 4

Preheat the oven to 350°F. Heat the oil in a heavy-based frying pan and brown the chicken in batches over medium heat. Drain on paper towels, then transfer to a casserole dish.

Add the garlic, onion and mushrooms to the pan and cook over medium heat for 5 minutes, or until soft. Add to the chicken with the thyme and tomatoes and crush the tomatoes with a wooden spoon. Season with freshly ground black pepper.

Combine the stock, wine and tomato paste and pour over the chicken. Cover and bake for 1¼ hours, or until the chicken is tender.

Meanwhile, cook the pasta in a large saucepan of boiling water for 10 minutes, or until *al dente*. Drain well. Serve with the chicken.

nutrition per serving: Energy 730 Cal; Fat 21.7 g; Saturated fat 6 g; Protein 59.9 g; Carbohydrate 71 g; Fiber 6.1 g; Cholesterol 217 mg

WILD RICE AND MIXED MUSHROOM PILAF

THIS EASY RECIPE CAN BE SERVED AS A VEGETARIAN MAIN MEAL OR SIDE DISH. FOR AN EVEN LOWER GI VERSION, YOU CAN SUBSTITUTE THE WILD RICE WITH COARSE BULGUR.

^{2}/$_3$ cup wild rice
1^1/$_2$ cups salt-reduced vegetable stock
1^1/$_2$ tbsp reduced-fat olive or canola oil margarine
1 large onion, finely chopped
2 garlic cloves, crushed
1^1/$_4$ cups basmati rice
10^1/$_2$ oz mixed mushrooms, sliced
1^1/$_2$ tbsp chopped thyme
1 fresh bay leaf

10^1/$_2$ oz canned chickpeas, rinsed and drained
handful baby spinach leaves
2 tbsp chopped flat-leaf (Italian) parsley
2 tbsp pine nuts, lightly toasted, to serve

PREP TIME: 20 MINUTES + 5 MINUTES STANDING
COOKING TIME: 50 MINUTES
SERVINGS: 4–6

Rinse the wild rice and cook in a saucepan with plenty of boiling water for 25 minutes—it will only be partially cooked after this time. Drain.

When the rice is nearly done, pour the stock into a large saucepan with 1^1/$_2$ cups water and bring to a boil. Reduce the heat to a simmer.

Meanwhile, melt the margarine in a large frying pan. Add the onion and garlic and cook for 3–4 minutes, or until the onion is softened but not browned. Add the basmati rice and stir until the rice grains are coated with margarine, then stir in the mushrooms.

Add the wild rice, stock, thyme and bay leaf. Bring to a boil while stirring, then reduce the heat, cover tightly with a lid and simmer for 15 minutes, or until the rice is tender and the stock has been absorbed.

Leave to stand for 5 minutes. Remove the bay leaf. Season with freshly ground black pepper, add the chickpeas, spinach leaves and parsley and fluff up the rice with a fork until well mixed and the spinach has wilted. Sprinkle with pine nuts and serve.

HINT:
• Try a mix of button, field and Swiss brown mushrooms.

nutrition per serving (6): Energy 506 Cal; Fat 13.3 g; Saturated fat 1.5 g; Protein 14.8 g; Carbohydrate 77 g; Fiber 9.3 g; Cholesterol 0 mg

SPICY CHICKEN BURGERS

about 1 lb lean ground chicken
4 spring onions (scallions), finely chopped
4 tbsp finely chopped cilantro leaves
2 garlic cloves, crushed
¼ tsp cayenne pepper
1 egg white, lightly beaten
1 tbsp olive or canola oil
1 lemon, halved

5½ oz tabouleh
  (see recipe on page 95)
4 wholegrain bread rolls, halved (see Hint)

PREP TIME: 10 MINUTES + 20 MINUTES
  REFRIGERATION
COOKING TIME: 10 MINUTES
SERVINGS: 4

Mix together the chicken, spring onion, cilantro, garlic, cayenne pepper and egg white and season with a little salt and freshly ground black pepper. Shape the mixture into four patties. Refrigerate for 20 minutes before cooking.

Heat the oil in a large non-stick frying pan over medium heat, add the patties and cook for about 5 minutes on each side, or until browned and cooked through.

Squeeze the lemon on the cooked patties and drain well on paper towels. Add the patties to the halved wholegrain buns and fill with the tabouleh.

HINT:
• The coarser the bread, the lower the GI.

THESE CHICKEN BURGERS ARE EASY TO
MAKE AND ARE A MUCH HEALTHIER
ALTERNATIVE TO REGULAR FAST-FOOD
BURGERS.

nutrition per serving: Energy 386 Cal
Fat 14.1 g
Saturated fat 2.5 g
Protein 20.4 g
Carbohydrate 40.4 g
Fiber 6.6 g
Cholesterol 98 mg

151

SWEET THINGS

STRAWBERRY AND BANANA ICE

THIS DESSERT IS A DELICIOUS ALTERNATIVE TO ICE CREAM AND SUITABLE FOR PEOPLE WHO ARE INTOLERANT TO DAIRY FOODS. IT PROVIDES ANTIOXIDANTS, FIBER AND MOST MINERALS.

10½ oz silken tofu, chopped
1⅓ cups strawberries, roughly chopped
2 just-ripe bananas, roughly chopped
¼ cup sucralose or ¼ cup sugar (see Hints)

PREP TIME: 15 MINUTES + FREEZING
COOKING TIME: NONE
SERVINGS: 4

Place the tofu, strawberries, bananas and sucralose or sugar in a blender or food processor and process until smooth.

Pour the mixture into a shallow cake pan and freeze for 3 hours, or until almost frozen. Break up roughly with a fork or a spoon, then transfer to a large bowl and beat until it has a smooth texture. Pour the mixture evenly into a suitable container, cover and freeze again, until quite firm.

Alternatively, freeze the blended mixture in an ice cream machine according to the manufacturer's instructions, until thick and creamy, then store in a covered container in the freezer.

Transfer to the refrigerator for about 30 minutes before serving to allow the ice to soften slightly. Scoop the ice into bowls to serve.

HINTS:
- Silken tofu is readily available in the refrigerated section of most supermarkets and health food shops. You can also buy it in long-life packets. Make sure you buy silken tofu as this type does not go lumpy.
- Many dietitians advise diabetics to use sucralose instead of sugar when cooking. The nutritional information below has been assessed using sucralose.
- If you use sugar instead of sucralose, the dessert will contain more calories and have a slightly higher GI. However, it will still remain in the low-GI range.

nutrition per serving: Energy 154 Cal; Fat 5.2 g; Saturated fat 0.7 g; Protein 10.8 g; Carbohydrate 14.2 g; Fiber 3.8 g; Cholesterol 0 mg

FROZEN FRUIT YOGURT

THIS SWEET TREAT IS A GOOD SOURCE OF CALCIUM AND FIBER AND IS NICE AS A DESSERT OR SNACK—TRY FREEZING SOME INTO POPSICLE MOLDS FOR HEALTHY TREATS ON HOT DAYS.

1 cup chopped, mixed, low-GI fresh fruit (apple, just-ripe banana, peach, apricot, orange)
1 cup low-fat plain unsweetened yogurt

PREP TIME: 5 MINUTES + 4 HOURS FREEZING
COOKING TIME: NONE
SERVINGS: 4

Put the mixed fruit in a blender, add the yogurt and purée. Pour the mixture into a freezer tray and freeze.

For a lighter texture, remove the mixture from the freezer, return to the blender and whip, then refreeze. Repeat once more.

HINTS:
• Serve with a low-GI fruit salad: apples, pears, plums, nectarines, peaches, strawberries, just-ripe banana, mango, citrus fruit.
• The nutrition will vary depending on the type/ratio of fruit used.

nutrition per serving: Energy 57 Cal; Fat 0.2 g; Saturated fat 0.7 g; Protein 4.2 g; Carbohydrate 8.5 g; Fiber 1 g; Cholesterol 3 mg

THIS LOW-FAT, LOW-GI DESSERT IS
LIGHT AND EASY TO MAKE. IT IS A NICE
ALTERNATIVE TO ICE CREAM OR
PUDDING AND IS PARTICULARLY
DELICIOUS DURING THE SUMMER
MONTHS.

nutrition per serving: Energy 168 Cal
Fat 0.7 g
Saturated fat 0.3 g
Protein 18.1 g
Carbohydrate 17.9 g
Fiber 2.6 g
Cholesterol 10 mg

RASPBERRY MOUSSE

3 tsp powdered gelatin
1 cup low-fat vanilla yogurt with no added
   sugar
4 egg whites
1¼ cups fresh raspberries, coarsely
   mashed
fresh raspberries and mint leaves, to serve

PREP TIME: 30 MINUTES + CHILLING
COOKING TIME: NONE
SERVINGS: 4–6

Sprinkle the gelatin over 1 tablespoon of water in a small heatproof bowl and leave until spongy. Put the bowl in a saucepan of just boiled water, off the heat (the water should come halfway up the bowl). Stir until dissolved. Cool.

Put the vanilla yogurt in a large bowl, then add the cooled gelatin and mix well.

Beat the egg whites until stiff peaks form, then fold through the yogurt mixture until just combined. Transfer half the mixture to a separate bowl and fold in the mashed raspberries.

Divide the raspberry mixture among four tall glasses, then top with the vanilla mixture. Refrigerate for several hours, or until set. Decorate with extra fresh raspberries and mint leaves.

HINT:
• You can make this with frozen berries, but remember to thaw them before you use them.

MANGO PASSIONFRUIT SORBET

You can use any combination of fruit in this recipe. This tangy sorbet provides a refreshing burst of vitamin C and a variety of antioxidants.

1 cup sucralose or 1 cup sugar (see Hints)
⅓ cup passionfruit pulp (about 8 passionfruit)
½ large mango, chopped
1 large peach, chopped
2 tbsp lemon juice
1 egg white

Prep time: 20 minutes + 8 hours freezing
Cooking time: 5 minutes
Servings: 6

Put the sucralose in a saucepan with 1 cup water. Stir over low heat until dissolved. Increase the heat, bring to a boil then transfer to a glass bowl, cool, then refrigerate. Strain the passionfruit pulp, reserving 1 tablespoon of the seeds.

Blend the fruit, passionfruit juice and lemon juice in a blender until smooth. With the motor running, add the cold sugar syrup and about ½ cup water. Stir in the passionfruit seeds. Freeze in a shallow container, stirring occasionally, for about 2–3 hours without allowing it to become solid.

Break up the icy mixture roughly with a fork or spoon, transfer to a bowl and beat with electric beaters to combine. (It should remain icy.) Beat the egg white in a small bowl until firm peaks form, then fold into the mixture until just combined. Freeze for up to 1 hour or serve at once. It will solidify if frozen for longer.

HINTS:
- If you are making the sorbet with sugar, in Step 2, freeze the mixture for up to 5 hours. In Step 3, beat the mixture until smooth and fluffy. Beat the egg white in a small bowl until firm peaks form, then fold into the mixture until just combined. Spread into a loaf tin and return to the freezer until firm. Transfer to the refrigerator, to soften, 15 minutes before serving. The sorbet will contain more calories if you use sugar.
- To make a berry sorbet, use 1 cup blackberries or blueberries, 1 cup hulled strawberries and 1 small peach. Prepare as above.

nutrition per serving: Energy 188 Cal; Fat 0.1 g; Saturated fat 0 g; Protein 1.6 g; Carbohydrate 44.7 g; Fiber 3 g; Cholesterol 0 mg

PEAR SORBET

THIS LOW-FAT, LOW-GI SORBET MAKES A REFRESHING DESSERT ON ITS OWN OR YOU CAN SERVE IT WITH SOME CANNED PEARS AND LOW-FAT YOGURT OR ICE CREAM.

about 4 lbs very ripe pears
1 cup sucralose or 2 cups sugar (see Hints)
1 cup water

PREP TIME: 40 MINUTES + OVERNIGHT FREEZING
COOKING TIME: 15 MINUTES
SERVINGS: 4–6

Thickly peel the pears, then core them and slice them into thick pieces. Place the pears in a large saucepan, just cover with water and simmer for about 10 minutes, or until tender. Drain and set aside to cool.

Purée the pears in a blender or food processor until smooth.

Combine the sucralose and water in a saucepan over medium heat and stir through. After the sucralose has completely dissolved, take the syrup off the stove and set aside to cool.

Mix together the syrup and pear purée, then pour into a shallow metal pan. Freeze until just solid.

Remove the pan from the freezer. Beat or process until a "slush" forms. Return to the pan and freeze until firm.

HINTS:
• Sorbets may be served before the main course to refresh the palate, or with other creams or fruit as a dessert.
• If you use sugar instead of sucralose the sorbet will contain more calories.

nutrition per serving: Energy 130 Cal; Fat 0.2 g; Saturated fat 0 g; Protein 0.6 g; Carbohydrate 30.8 g; Fiber 3.7 g; Cholesterol 0 mg

SUMMER FRUITY YOGURT

2 ripe pears, unpeeled
2 tsp lemon juice
½ cup fresh or frozen blueberries
1¼ cups strawberries, hulled, halved and
    quartered
pulp of 2 passionfruit
1 tbsp sucralose or sugar (see Hints)

2 cups low-fat vanilla or fruit-flavored
    yogurt, sweetened with a low-calorie
    sweetener
⅓ cup raw pistachio kernels, chopped

PREP TIME: 10 MINUTES + CHILLING TIME
COOKING TIME: NONE
SERVINGS: 4

Remove the core from the pears. Cut into chunks and put into a large bowl, sprinkle with the lemon juice. Add the blueberries, strawberries and passionfruit and sprinkle with the sucralose or sugar. Set aside for 10 minutes to infuse. Gently fold through the yogurt until it is just lightly coating the fruit.

Spoon into four 1 cup parfait glasses and chill for at least 20 minutes. Sprinkle with the pistachios, and serve.

HINTS:
• For variety you can also make this recipe with raspberries, nectarines or peaches, or chopped citrus fruits.
• Using 1 tablespoon sugar instead of sucralose will increase the energy content and GI of this dessert, but it will still be low GI.
• Low-fat yogurt that is sweetened with a low-calorie sweetener, instead of sugar, has less energy and a lower GI than sugar-sweetened low-fat yogurt. Compare the sugar and energy values on yogurt containers to find non-sugar sweetened varieties.

THIS LIGHT DESSERT IS GREAT IN SUMMER,
BUT IT CAN BE ENJOYED AT ANY TIME OF YEAR
USING THE LOW-GI FRUIT THAT'S IN SEASON. IT
TAKES LITTLE TIME TO PREPARE AND IS STYLISH
ENOUGH TO SERVE AT A CASUAL DINNER PARTY.

nutrition per serving: Energy 213 Cal
Fat 6.8 g
Saturated fat 0.8 g
Protein 11.1 g
Carbohydrate 23.6 g
Fiber 5.7 g
Cholesterol 10 mg

161

FRUIT JELLIES

THESE LOW-GI HOMEMADE FRUIT JELLIES CONTAIN NO ARTIFICIAL COLORS OR FLAVORS. THE BERRIES PROVIDE SOME FIBER, FOLATE AND ANTIOXIDANTS.

4 tsp gelatin
2 cups cranberry and raspberry juice
1½ cups mixed berries, fresh or frozen

PREP TIME: 20 MINUTES + REFRIGERATION
COOKING TIME: NONE
SERVINGS: 4

Sprinkle the gelatin in an even layer onto 3 tablespoons of the juice, in a small bowl, and leave to go spongy. Bring a small pan of water to a boil, remove from the heat and place the bowl in the pan. The water should come halfway up the side of the bowl. Stir the gelatin until clear and dissolved. Cool slightly and mix with the rest of the juice.

Rinse four ¾ cup molds with water (wet molds make it easier when unmolding) and pour ¾ in of the juice into each. Refrigerate until set.

Meanwhile, if the fruit is frozen, defrost it and add any liquid to the remaining juice. When the bottom layer of jelly has set, divide the fruit among the molds (reserving a few berries to garnish) and divide the rest of the juice among the molds, pouring it over the fruit. Refrigerate until set.

To turn out the jellies, hold each mold in a hot, damp dish towel and turn out onto a plate. Ease away the edge of the jelly with your finger to break the seal. (If you turn the jellies onto a damp plate you will be able to move them around, otherwise they will stick.) Garnish with the reserved berries.

nutrition per serving: Energy 84 Cal; Fat 0.1 g; Saturated fat 0 g; Protein 4.3 g; Carbohydrate 15.5 g; Fiber 1.9 g; Cholesterol 0 mg

SPICED POACHED PEARS

ENJOY THE DELICATE FLAVORS OF THIS LOW-FAT DESSERT. THE PEARS ARE EASILY DIGESTED AND PROVIDE POTASSIUM AND SOLUBLE FIBER. SERVE THEM WITH YOGURT FOR EXTRA PROTEIN, CALCIUM AND PHOSPHORUS.

6 beurre bosc pears
1¼ cups rosé wine (see Hint)
¾ cup pure apple or pear juice
4 cloves
1 vanilla bean, halved
1 cinnamon stick
1 tbsp pure maple syrup

7 oz low-fat vanilla yogurt sweetened with a low-calorie sweetener

PREP TIME: 10 MINUTES + 30 MINUTES
   STANDING
COOKING TIME: 20 MINUTES
SERVINGS: 6

Peel, halve and core the pears. Place in a deep frying pan with a lid, and add the wine or water, fruit juice and cloves. Scrape the seeds out of the vanilla bean and add both the seeds and pod to the pan. Stir in the cinnamon stick and maple syrup. Bring to a boil, then reduce the heat and simmer for 5–7 minutes, or until the pears are tender. Remove from the heat and cover with the lid.

Leave the fruit for 30 minutes to allow the flavors to infuse, then remove the pears with a slotted spoon and place in a serving dish. Return the syrup to the heat and boil for 6–8 minutes, or until reduced by half. Strain the syrup over the pears. Serve warm or chilled with the yogurt.

HINT:
• If you'd prefer not to use wine, the same amount of liquid can be replaced with additional apple and pear juice.

nutrition per serving: Energy 174 Cal; Fat 0.3 g; Saturated fat 0.04 g; Protein 2.5 g; Carbohydrate 32.4 g; Fiber 3.4 g; Cholesterol 3 mg

THIS NEW VERSION OF BREAD AND BUTTER
PUDDING HAS LESS FAT AND BREAD AND MORE
CUSTARD THAN USUAL, GIVING THE PUDDING A
SOFTER TEXTURE. IT IS A GREAT WINTER DESSERT
BUT IT ISN'T LOW IN CALORIES—SO ENJOY IN
MODERATION.

nutrition per serving: Energy 169 Cal
Fat 3.1 g
Saturated fat 0.8 g
Protein 8.9 g
Carbohydrate 25.2 g
Fiber 3.2 g
Cholesterol 65 mg

BAKED FRUIT BREAD CUSTARD

4 slices low-GI wholegrain fruit bread
1 tbsp sugar-free marmalade spread
½ cup chopped dried peaches
2 eggs
1 egg white
¼ cup sucralose or ¼ cup sugar (see Hints)
1 tsp grated lemon zest

2 cups low-fat milk
freshly grated nutmeg, to sprinkle

PREP TIME: 15 MINUTES
COOKING TIME: 35 MINUTES
SERVINGS: 6

Preheat the oven to 325°F. Spread the bread slices with the marmalade spread, cut each bread slice into quarters and arrange in a 5-cup ceramic baking dish. Scatter with the chopped peaches.

Whisk together the eggs, egg white, sucralose or sugar and lemon zest in a bowl. Whisk in the milk. Pour over the bread and sprinkle with nutmeg. Set aside for 5 minutes to allow the bread to soften.

Put the dish in a roasting tin of hot water. The water should come halfway up the sides of the dish. Bake for 35 minutes, or until set. Serve with low-fat ice cream or low-fat yogurt.

HINTS:
• If you use sugar instead of sucralose, the dessert will contain more calories and have a slightly higher GI. However, it will still remain in the low-GI range.
• There are many different types of fruit bread on the market and not all of them are low GI so you will need to read the label carefully.

DRIED APRICOT FOOL

THIS LOW-FAT FRUIT DESSERT IS RICH IN POTASSIUM AND BETACAROTENE. IT IS A GOOD SOURCE OF FIBER AND PROVIDES A LITTLE IRON. IT SHOULD ONLY BE AN OCCASSIONAL TREAT THOUGH AS IT IS NOT LOW IN CALORIES.

1 oz finely chopped candied ginger
6 oz dried apricots, chopped
2 egg whites
2 tbsp sucralose or 2 tbsp caster sugar
1 tbsp shredded coconut, toasted

PREP TIME: 15 MINUTES
COOKING TIME: 5 MINUTES
SERVINGS: 4

Place the ginger, apricots and 4 tablespoons water in a small saucepan. Cook, covered, over very low heat for 5 minutes, stirring occasionally. Remove from the heat and allow to cool completely.

Using electric beaters, beat the egg whites in a clean, dry bowl until soft peaks form. Add the sucralose or sugar and beat until just combined. Quickly and gently fold the cooled apricot mixture into the egg mixture and divide among four chilled serving glasses. Scatter the toasted coconut over the top and serve immediately.

HINTS:
• When adding the sucralose, be sure not to beat it for too long as it can clump and be difficult to fold.
• The apricots can scorch easily, so cook over low heat. Serve immediately, or the egg white will slowly break down and lose volume.
• If you use sugar instead of sucralose, the dessert will contain more calories and have a slightly higher GI. However, it will still remain in the low-GI range.

nutrition per serving: Energy 136 Cal; Fat 1.1 g; Saturated fat 0.9 g; Protein 3.7 g; Carbohydrate 26.1 g; Fiber 4.3 g; Cholesterol 0 mg

STONE-FRUIT SALAD

A COLORFUL, REFRESHING DESSERT, BASED ON LOW-GI FRUIT, THAT'S QUICK AND EASY TO MAKE, AND A RICH SOURCE OF ANTIOXIDANTS.

4 apricots, unpeeled, halved and thinly sliced

4 peaches, unpeeled, halved and thinly sliced

4 nectarines, unpeeled, halved and thinly sliced

4 plums, unpeeled, halved and thinly sliced

2 tbsp unsweetened apricot juice or nectar

7 oz light vanilla yogurt

PREP TIME: 15 MINUTES

COOKING TIME: NONE

SERVINGS: 4

Mix the fruit together and drizzle with apricot juice. Serve the fruit salad with the fromage frais dessert.

HINT:
• You can replace the yogurt with low-fat ice cream, if you prefer.

nutrition per serving: Energy 211 Cal; Fat 0.7 g; Saturated fat 0.1 g; Protein 8 g; Carbohydrate 36.3 g; Fiber 8.2 g; Cholesterol 3 mg

APPLE AND STRAWBERRY CRUMBLE

28 oz canned unsweetened apple pie filling

1$\frac{2}{3}$ cups strawberries, hulled and sliced

$\frac{3}{4}$ cup wholegrain rolled oats

$\frac{1}{4}$ cup sucralose or $\frac{1}{4}$ cup brown sugar (see Hint)

$\frac{1}{4}$ cup stoneground, whole-wheat, all-purpose flour

1 tbsp pumpkin seeds

1$\frac{1}{2}$ tbsp cold, reduced-fat olive or canola oil margarine

low-fat, sugar-free vanilla or strawberry yogurt, to serve

PREP TIME: 10 MINUTES

COOKING TIME: 20 MINUTES

SERVINGS: 6

Preheat the oven to 350°F. Place the apples in a 6 x 8 x 2 in ovenproof dish. Stir through the strawberries.

Combine the rolled oats, sucralose or brown sugar, flour and pumpkin seeds in a bowl. Rub in the margarine, using the fingertips, until crumbly. Do not overmix. Spread evenly over the apple. Bake for 20 minutes, or until golden brown. Serve with the yogurt.

HINT:

• If you use brown sugar instead of sucralose, the dessert will contain more calories and have a slightly higher GI. However, it will still remain in the low-GI range.

THIS DESSERT DELIVERS EVERYTHING
YOU WANT IN A CRUMBLE WITH LESS
FAT AND CALORIES THAN TRADITIONAL
FRUIT CRUMBLES.

nutrition per serving: Energy 191 Cal
Fat 5.3 g
Saturated fat 1.7 g
Protein 3.8 g
Carbohydrate 30 g
Fiber 4.9
Cholesterol 0 mg

ORANGE SEMOLINA CAKE

EVERYONE NEEDS SOMETHING SWEET NOW AND THEN AND THIS CAKE IS A GREAT CHOICE FOR AN OCCASIONAL TREAT. IT IS LOW GI, BUT IT IS STILL A HIGH CALORIE TREAT, SO ENJOY IN MODERATION.

olive or canola oil spray
1 cup stoneground, self-rising flour
1 cup semolina
½ cup ground almonds
⅓ cup sucralose or ⅓ cup raw sugar (see Hints)
3 eggs
3 tbsp reduced-fat olive or canola oil margarine, just melted
1 cup buttermilk

2 tbsp orange juice
1 tbsp grated orange zest

PREP TIME: 20 MINUTES
COOKING TIME: 50 MINUTES
SERVINGS: 8–10

Preheat the oven to 325°F. Lightly spray a 8 in round cake pan with oil, then line the base with baking paper.

Sift the flour into a large bowl, add the semolina, ground almonds and sucralose, then return any husks to the bowl. Mix together and make a well in the center.

Put the eggs, margarine, buttermilk, orange juice and orange zest in a bowl and whisk until well combined. Stir into the flour mixture and mix until smooth. Spoon into the prepared pan and smooth the surface.

Bake for 45–50 minutes, or until cooked when tested with a metal skewer. Leave in the pan for 10 minutes, then turn out onto a wire rack to cool completely (you may need to gently loosen the cake from the tin with a knife). Serve in wedges with some berries, stone fruit or orange slices and low-fat yogurt.

HINTS:
• The cake will keep refrigerated for up to 1 week. Freeze for up to 1 month.
• If you are using raw sugar, this will raise the cake's GI into the medium-GI range. It will also contain more calories.

nutrition per serving (10): Energy 188 Cal; Fat 7.8 g; Saturated fat 1.4 g; Protein 6.9 g; Carbohydrate 21.7 g; Fiber 1.5 g; Cholesterol 59 mg

FRUITY LAYER CAKE

THIS DELICIOUS, MOIST CAKE CONTAINS FEWER CALORIES THAN TRADITIONAL FRUIT CAKE AND IS STYLISH ENOUGH TO SERVE AT A SPECIAL OCCASION OR BAKE AS A GIFT FOR A FRIEND. ALTHOUGH LOW GI, THIS CAKE IS ENERGY-DENSE SO ENJOY ONE SLICE AS AN OCCASIONAL TREAT.

1 large green apple, peeled, cored and chopped
⅓ cup chopped pitted prunes
⅓ cup chopped dried apricots
⅓ cup chopped dried peaches or dried pears
½ tsp ground cinnamon
olive or canola oil spray
3 tbsp reduced-fat olive or canola oil margarine
½ cup sucralose or ½ cup brown sugar
2 eggs

1⅓ cups stoneground, whole-wheat, self-rising flour
¼ cup desiccated coconut
2 tbsp unprocessed oat bran
¾ cup low-fat milk

PREP TIME: 25 MINUTES
COOKING TIME: 1 HOUR
SERVINGS: 10–12

To make the filling, put the chopped apple, prunes, apricots and peaches and cinnamon in a saucepan with ½ cup water. Cover and cook over low heat for 10–15 minutes, or until the fruit has softened and the water has been absorbed. Cool.

Preheat the oven to 350°F. Spray a deep, 8 in square cake pan with oil, then line the base with baking paper.

To make the cake batter, put the margarine and sucralose or brown sugar in a bowl and beat with electric beaters for 1 minute. Add the eggs one at a time, beating well after each addition. (If using sucralose the mixture will look curdled.)

Fold the combined sifted flour, including any husks, coconut and oat bran into the batter alternating with the milk. Spread half the batter over the base of the prepared pan. Spoon over the cooled fruit and roughly spoon the remaining batter over the fruit. There will be gaps of fruit showing.

Bake for 45 minutes, or until a skewer inserted in the center comes out clean, and the cake is lightly golden brown on top. Cool in the pan for 10 minutes, then turn out onto a wire rack to cool. Serve warm or cold.

nutrition per serving (12): Energy 155 Cal; Fat 4.7 g; Saturated fat 1.9 g; Protein 4.8 g; Carbohydrate 21.4 g; Fiber 4.1 g; Cholesterol 32 mg

THIS SWEET BREAD HAS A DELICIOUS
FLAVOR COMBINATION THAT IS GREAT AT ANY
TIME OF DAY. YOU CAN FREEZE INDIVIDUAL
SLICES OF THIS LOAF TO PACK INTO
LUNCHBOXES OR PICNIC BASKETS.

nutrition per serving: Energy 197 Cal
Fat 10.7 g
Saturated fat 1.2 g
Protein 4.6 g
Carbohydrate 20 g
Fiber 1.7 g
Cholesterol 31 mg

ZUCCHINI AND PISTACHIO LOAF

olive or canola oil spray

1 cup stoneground, self-rising flour

½ tsp freshly grated nutmeg

½ tsp baking soda

¾ cup semolina

¼ cup brown sugar (or half sucralose, see Hints)

½ cup raw pistachio nuts, chopped

2 eggs

⅓ cup unsweetened apple purée

4 tbs olive or canola oil

2 tsp grated lemon or lime zest

1 cup grated zucchini

PREP TIME: 20 MINUTES

COOKING TIME: 50 MINUTES

MAKES 10–12 SLICES

Preheat the oven to 325°F. Spray an 8 x 4 in loaf pan with oil, then line the base with baking paper.

Sift the flour, nutmeg and baking soda into a large bowl, then return any husks to the bowl. Stir in the semolina, brown sugar and pistachio nuts. Make a well in the center.

Whisk together the eggs, apple purée, oil and lemon zest in a bowl. Squeeze out any excess moisture from the grated zucchini, then stir into the egg mixture. Add all at once to the flour mixture and stir until combined and smooth. Spoon into the prepared pan and smooth the surface.

Bake for 45–50 minutes, or until cooked when tested with a metal skewer. Leave in the pan for 10 minutes, then turn out onto a wire rack to cool completely. Cut into slices to serve.

HINTS:
- You can replace half the sugar with sucralose if you prefer. The sucralose will lower the GI and calorie content of the loaf, which is good if you have diabetes or are watching your weight.
- You will need 2 medium zucchini to yield 1 cup grated.
- The loaf will keep refrigerated for up to 1 week and can be stored frozen for up to 1 month.

MIXED FRUIT AND BANANA BREAD

THE DRIED FRUIT IN THIS NEW VERSION OF BANANA BREAD PACKS A LOT OF FLAVOR INTO EACH SLICE. THIS LOW-GI BREAD IS MORE NUTRITIOUS THAN MANY CAKES AND COOKIES, BUT SHOULD STILL BE ENJOYED IN MODERATION AS AN OCCASIONAL TREAT.

olive or canola oil spray
$1^2/_3$ cups stoneground,
   self-rising flour
1 tsp baking powder
1 tsp pumpkin pie spice
$3^1/_2$ oz chopped dried pears
$3^1/_2$ oz chopped dried peaches
$1/_4$ cup natural oat bran
$1/_3$ cup sucralose or $1/_3$ cup sugar (see Hints)
$1/_2$ cup hazelnuts, roughly chopped
   (optional)

2 eggs
$1^1/_4$ cups plain low-fat yogurt
3 tbsp canola oil
1 large just-ripe banana, mashed

PREP TIME: 20 MINUTES
COOKING TIME: 50 MINUTES
MAKES 10–12 SLICES

Preheat the oven to 325°F. Spray a 9 x 5 in loaf pan with oil, then line the base with baking paper.

Sift the flour, baking powder and mixed spice into a large bowl, then return any husks to the bowl. Stir in the dried pears and peaches and use your hands to mix and separate the chopped fruit. Stir in the oat bran, sucralose or sugar and chopped hazelnuts.

Whisk together the eggs, yogurt, oil and mashed banana in a bowl. Add to the flour mixture and stir until combined and smooth. Spoon into the prepared pan and smooth the surface.

Bake for 50 minutes, or until a skewer inserted in the center comes out clean. Cover with foil for the last 10 minutes if it is browning too much. Leave in the pan for 15 minutes, then turn out onto a wire rack to cool. Cut into slices to serve. Serve warm or cold. Delicious toasted.

HINTS:
• Using sugar instead of sucralose will increase the bread's GI and calorie content, but the bread will remain in the low-GI range.
• Will keep refrigerated for up to 1 week. Freeze for up to 1 month.
• Eat it as a treat only as the hazelnuts are quite high in fat. If preferred, you can leave them out.

nutrition per serving (12): Energy 237 Cal; Fat 9.6 g; Saturated fat 0.8 g; Protein 6.7 g; Carbohydrate 29.1 g; Fiber 3.6 g; Cholesterol 33 mg

CARROT WALNUT LOAF

THIS IS A HEALTHIER CHOICE THAN COMMERCIAL CARROT CAKE OR CHOCOLATE CAKE BUT IT'S NOT LOW IN CALORIES.

olive or canola oil spray
1 cup stoneground, self-rising flour
½ tsp baking soda
1 tsp ground cinnamon
¾ cup coarse semolina
⅓ cup sucralose or ⅓ cup raw sugar (see Hints)
½ cup walnuts, chopped
½ cup dried-fruit medley
1½ cups grated carrot

2 eggs
1 cup buttermilk
4 tbsp olive or canola oil

PREP TIME: 20 MINUTES
COOKING TIME: 50 MINUTES
MAKES 10–12 SLICES

Preheat the oven to 325°F. Spray an 8 x 4 in loaf pan with oil, then line the base with baking paper.

Sift the flour, baking soda and cinnamon into a large bowl, then return any husks to the bowl. Stir in the semolina and sucralose or raw sugar, then stir in the walnuts, fruit medley and grated carrot. Make a well in the center.

Whisk together the eggs, buttermilk and oil in a bowl. Add to the flour mixture and stir until combined and smooth. Spoon into the prepared pan and smooth the surface.

Bake for 50 minutes, or until a skewer inserted in the center comes out clean. Leave in the pan for 10 minutes, then turn out onto a wire rack to cool completely. Cut into slices to serve.

HINTS:
• Using raw sugar instead of sucralose will increase the loaf's GI and calorie content, but the loaf will remain in the low-GI range.
• Will keep refrigerated for up to 1 week and frozen for up to 1 month.
• Fruit medley is a mixture of dried apple, apricots, pears and raisins.

nutrition per serving (12): Energy 203 Cal; Fat 11.1 g; Saturated fat 1.2 g; Protein 5 g; Carbohydrate 19.8 g; Fiber 2.1 g; Cholesterol 33 mg

LEMON BERRY CHEESECAKE

FRUITY BASE
2¼ oz dried apricots
2¼ oz dried pitted dates
2¼ oz dried figs
⅓ cup coarse semolina

CHEESECAKE
10½ oz low-fat ricotta cheese
2 tbsp sucralose or 2 tbsp sugar (see Hint)
9 oz low-fat, French vanilla, Greek-style yogurt

9 oz low-fat, Greek-style, lemon-flavored yogurt
2 tsp finely grated lemon zest
2 tbsp lemon juice
1 tbsp gelatin
2 egg whites
9 oz strawberries, halved

PREP TIME: 25 MINUTES + OVERNIGHT REFRIGERATION
COOKING TIME: NONE
SERVINGS: 12

Lightly oil and line the base and side of an 8 in spring-form cake pan with plastic wrap. Line the base, over the plastic, with baking paper. Process the dried fruit in a food processor until finely chopped; add the semolina and blend well together. Use fingers to spread evenly over the base of the prepared pan. Refrigerate.

Combine the ricotta and sucralose or sugar in a food processor until smooth. Add all the yogurt, the lemon zest and juice, then mix well. Transfer to a large bowl.

Put 3 tablespoons of water in a small bowl, sprinkle the gelatin in an even layer onto the surface and leave to go spongy. Bring a small saucepan of water to a boil, remove from the heat and put the gelatin bowl in the pan. The water should come halfway up the side of the bowl. Stir the gelatin until clear and dissolved, then cool slightly. Stir the gelatin mixture into the ricotta mixture.

Beat the egg whites until soft peaks form, then gently fold into the ricotta mixture. Pour the mixture into the pan evenly over the fruity base and refrigerate for several hours or overnight, until set. Carefully remove from the pan by removing the side of the pan and easing the plastic from the sides. Use a spatula to aid in lifting the cheesecake off the baking paper, removing the plastic wrap. Put on a serving platter and decorate with the halved strawberries.

HINT:
• Using sugar instead of sucralose will increase the GI and calorie content, but the cheesecake will remain in the low-GI range.

THIS TANGY, LOW-FAT CHEESECAKE
PROVIDES SOME BETACAROTENE,
CALCIUM AND PHOSPHORUS.

nutrition per serving: Energy 134 Cal
Protein 8.8 g
Fat 1.5 g
Saturated fat 0.6 g
Carbohydrate 19.6 g
Fiber 2.3 g
Cholesterol 2 mg

177

WHOLEMEAL APRICOT COOKIES

DELICIOUS SERVED WARM OR COLD, THESE CRUNCHY COOKIES WILL QUICKLY BECOME A FAMILY FAVORITE. THEY MAKE A NICE TREAT TO TAKE ALONG TO PICNICS.

1½ cups stoneground, self-rising flour

1 tsp baking powder

1½ tsp ground cinnamon

¼ cup shredded coconut

¼ cup unprocessed oat bran

⅓ cup sucralose or ⅓ cup raw sugar (see Hints)

3 tbsp cold, reduced-fat olive or canola oil margarine

1 cup dried apricots, chopped

1 tbsp sunflower or pumpkin seeds

1 egg

4 tbsp low-fat milk

PREP TIME: 20 MINUTES

COOKING TIME: 20 MINUTES

MAKES 24

Preheat the oven to 350°F. Line a large baking tray with baking paper.

Sift the flour, baking powder and cinnamon into a large bowl, then return any husks to the bowl. Stir in the coconut, oat bran and sucralose or raw sugar. Using clean fingers, rub the margarine into the mixture until crumbly. Stir in the apricots and seeds. Make a well in the center.

Combine the egg and milk in a small bowl. Pour into the well in the dry ingredients and mix briefly with a fork until just combined into a rough dough.

Using 1 heaped tablespoon of mixture at a time, put spoonfuls onto the tray, forming a little mound, then flatten slightly. Bake for 15–20 minutes, or until cooked and golden brown—watching carefully that they don't burn. Leave on the tray for 2–3 minutes then transfer to a wire rack to cool completely.

HINTS:
• Store in an airtight container for up to 5 days.
• Using sugar instead of sucralose will increase the cookies' GI and calorie content, but they will remain in the low-GI range.

nutrition per cookie (24): Energy 81 Cal; Fat 2.6 g; Saturated fat 1.0 g; Protein 2.1 g; Carbohydrate 11.5 g; Fiber 1.6 g; Cholesterol 8 mg

HAZELNUT BROWNIES

KIDS AND ADULTS WILL LOVE THIS CRUNCHY TREAT, AND BEING SMALL THEY ARE EASY TO TAKE TO PICNICS, BARBECUES AND ON CAMPING TRIPS. FOR VARIETY AND EXTRA OMEGA-3 FAT, YOU CAN REPLACE THE HAZELNUTS WITH PECANS OR WALNUTS.

olive or canola oil spray
1 cup stoneground, self-rising flour
½ cup cocoa powder
½ teaspoon baking soda
1¼ cups sucralose or 1¼ cups raw sugar (see Hints)
⅓ cup dark chocolate chips
½ cup raw hazelnuts, roughly chopped
2 eggs
1 cup buttermilk
¼ cup unsweetened apple sauce

2 tbsp olive or canola oil
1 tsp natural vanilla extract
confectioners' sugar, to dust

PREP TIME: 15 MINUTES
COOKING TIME: 40 MINUTES
MAKES 14–16 SQUARES

Preheat the oven to 350°F. Spray a 11 x 7 in shallow baking tin with oil, then line the base with baking paper overhanging the two long sides.

Sift the flour, cocoa and baking soda into a large bowl, then return any husks to the bowl. Stir in the sucralose or raw sugar then the chocolate chips and hazelnuts. Make a well in the center.

Whisk together the eggs, buttermilk, apple sauce, oil and vanilla in a bowl. Add to the flour mixture and stir until just combined and smooth. Do not overmix. Pour into the prepared pan and smooth the surface.

Bake for 40 minutes, or until a skewer inserted in the center comes out clean. Leave in the tin for 10 minutes, then turn out onto a wire rack to cool completely. Dust with confectioners' sugar and cut into squares to serve.

HINTS:
• Store in an airtight container for up to 5 days.
• People with diabetes should make this recipe with sucralose rather than sugar because sugar will increase this recipe's calorie content and GI.

nutrition per square (16): Energy 143 Cal; Fat 7.6 g; Saturated fat 1.7 g; Protein 4 g; Carbohydrate 13.9 g; Fiber 1.1 g; Cholesterol 25 mg

THIS RECIPE IS QUICK AND EASY TO MAKE AND IS SUITABLE FOR THE WHOLE FAMILY AS A SPECIAL TREAT. THE OATS MAKE THIS SLICE MORE FILLING TO HELP YOU FEEL SATISFIED WITH JUST ONE PIECE.

nutrition per serving (16): Energy 139 Cal
Fat 7.3 g
Saturated fat 2 g
Protein 3.3 g
Carbohydrate 14.2 g
Fiber 2.3 g
Cholesterol 0.5 mg

180

CHOCOLATE FRUIT AND NUT SLICE

olive or canola oil spray

1 cup stoneground, whole-wheat, self-rising flour

2 tbsp unsweetened cocoa powder

½ cup wholegrain rolled oats

⅓ cup shredded coconut

2 tbsp unprocessed oat bran

⅓ cup sucralose or ⅓ cup brown sugar (see Hints)

½ cup dried-fruit medley, chopped

½ cup walnuts, chopped

½ cup reduced-fat canola oil margarine, just melted

1 tbsp pure maple syrup

1 cup low-fat milk

confectioners' sugar, to dust

PREP TIME: 15 MINUTES

COOKING TIME: 25 MINUTES

MAKES 14–16 SLICES

Preheat the oven to 350°F. Spray an 11 x 7 in shallow baking pan with oil, then line the base with baking paper overhanging the two long sides.

Sift the flour and cocoa into a large bowl, then return any husks to the bowl. Stir in the rolled oats, coconut, oat bran and sucralose or brown sugar, fruit medley and walnuts. Make a well in the center.

Combine the melted margarine, maple syrup and milk in a small bowl. Add to the flour mixture and stir until well combined. Spread evenly into the prepared pan.

Bake for 25 minutes, or until cooked and firm. Leave in the tin to cool, then turn out onto a wire rack to cool completely. Dust with confectioners' sugar and cut into slices to serve. Delicious served with berries and low-fat yogurt or berry fromage frais.

HINTS:
• Will keep in an airtight container for 5 days. Freeze for up to 1 month.
• Replace walnuts with pecans if liked.
• If you have diabetes, this recipe is best made with sucralose or another low-calorie sugar substitute instead of sugar because sugar will increase the slice's calorie content and effect on your blood sugar level.

GLUTEN-FREE PEAR MUFFINS

HOMEMADE MUFFINS LIKE THESE ARE EASY TO MAKE. FREE OF GLUTEN, NUTS AND SOY, THEY CAN ALSO BE MADE WITH OTHER FRUIT COMBINATIONS.

olive or canola oil, for greasing

2 cups soy-free, gluten-free, self-rising flour

2 tsp gluten-free baking powder

¾ cup sucralose or ¾ cup brown sugar (see Hints)

⅔ cup low-fat milk

4 tbsp olive or canola oil

2 eggs, or equivalent egg replacer

2 ripe pears (about 1 lb), peeled, cored and mashed

PREP TIME: 15 MINUTES

COOKING TIME: 20 MINUTES

MAKES 12

Preheat the oven to 350°F. Lightly grease a muffin pan with oil.

Sift the flour and baking powder into a large bowl and add the sucralose or brown sugar. In a separate bowl, combine the milk, oil and eggs or egg replacer. Add the milk mixture and pears to the flour mixture. Use a large spoon to mix until just combined. Spoon the mixture into the muffin pan.

Bake for 18–20 minutes, or until a skewer inserted in the center comes out clean. Leave for 5 minutes before turning onto a wire rack.

HINTS:
• These muffins need to be eaten the day they are made.
• Using sugar instead of sucralose will increase the muffins' GI and calorie content but they will remain in the low- to medium-GI range.

nutrition per muffin: Energy 168 Cal; Fat 7.1 g; Saturated fat 0.7 g; Protein 2 g; Carbohydrate 24 g; Fiber 2.7 g; Cholesterol 32 mg

BERRY MUFFINS

THESE TANGY MUFFINS ARE PERFECT, SERVED WARM OR COLD, FOR BREAKFAST, BRUNCH OR
AFTERNOON TEA. THE BUTTERMILK ADDS FLAVOR AND LIGHTENS THE TEXTURE. THEY ARE NOT LOW
IN CALORIES, SO ENJOY IN MODERATION.

olive or canola oil spray
1¼ cups stoneground, self-rising flour
1 tsp baking powder
1 tsp ground cinnamon
¼ cup natural oat bran
½ cup wholegrain rolled oats
⅓ cup sucralose or ⅓ cup sugar (see Hints)
1 cup blueberries, frozen or fresh
½ cup raspberries, frozen or fresh
1 egg

2 cups buttermilk
3 tbsp reduced-fat canola oil margarine,
   just melted
1 tsp natural vanilla extract
confectioners' sugar, to dust

PREP TIME: 20 MINUTES
COOKING TIME: 25 MINUTES
MAKES 12

Preheat the oven to 350°F. Spray muffin pan with oil.

Sift the flour, baking powder and cinnamon into a large bowl, then return any husks to the
bowl. Stir in the oat bran, rolled oats, sucralose or sugar and berries. Make a well in the
center.

Whisk together the egg, buttermilk, melted margarine and vanilla and stir into the flour
mixture until just combined. Do not overmix. Spoon evenly into the muffin pan.

Bake for 25 minutes, or until firm to touch. Leave in the pan for 5 minutes, then turn out
onto a wire rack to cool. Dust with confectioners' sugar and serve warm or cold with fresh
berries.

HINTS:
• Will keep refrigerated for up to 5 days or frozen for up to 1 month.
• These muffins can also be made in a mini muffin pan to produce small treats that can be
  added to a packed lunch.
• Using sugar instead of sucralose will increase the muffins' calorie content and GI value
  into the medium-GI category.

nutrition per muffin: Energy 147 Cal; Fat 4.4 g; Saturated fat 1.2 g; Protein 4.7 g; Carbohydrate 20.6 g;
Fiber 2 g; Cholesterol 19 mg

FRUIT AND OAT BRAN MUFFINS

olive or canola oil spray

1½ cups stoneground, self-rising flour

1 tsp freshly grated nutmeg

½ tsp baking powder

1 cup unprocessed oat bran

⅓ cup sucralose or ⅓ cup raw sugar (see Hints)

1 cup dried-fruit medley

1 egg

1¼ cups low-fat milk

½ cup unsweetened apple sauce

3 tbsp reduced-fat olive or canola oil margarine, just melted

PREP TIME: 20 MINUTES

COOKING TIME: 25 MINUTES

MAKES 12

Preheat the oven to 350°F. Spray a muffin pan with oil.

Sift the flour, nutmeg and the baking powder into a large bowl, then return any husks to the bowl. Stir in the oat bran, sucralose or raw sugar and fruit medley, using your fingertips to break up the fruit medley so it doesn't clump together. Make a well in the center.

Whisk together the egg, milk, apple sauce and melted margarine and stir into the flour mixture until just combined. Do not overmix. Spoon evenly into the muffin pan.

Bake for 25 minutes, or until firm to the touch and golden brown. Leave in the pan for 5 minutes, then turn out onto a wire rack to cool.

HINTS:
• If you use sugar instead of sucralose the muffins will contain more calories and be low- to medium-GI.
• To lower the GI further and add some healthy omega-3 fat, you can substitute 3 tablespoons of the flour with ground linseed (flaxseed) meal. This may reduce the cooking time a little, so check the muffins from 20 minutes on.
• Will keep refrigerated for up to 5 days and frozen for up to 1 month.

THESE TASTY MUFFINS ARE A HEALTHY LOWER FAT ALTERNATIVE TO COMMERCIAL BRAN MUFFINS. HOWEVER, THEY ARE NOT LOW IN CALORIES, SO ENJOY IN MODERATION.

nutrition per muffin: Energy 181 Cal
Fat 4 g
Saturated fat 0.8 g
Protein 5.7 g
Carbohydrate 28.8 g
Fiber 3.6 g
Cholesterol 16 mg

SHOPPING LIST

bread

Bread and English muffins
with lots of grains in them
Pumpernickel bread (black
bread)
Sourdough bread—
wholegrain, rye, or
wholemeal
Fruit and spice loaf

breakfast cereals

Extruded bran cereals (not
bran flakes)
Semolina
Oatmeal made from
wholegrain, traditional rolled
oats, steel-cut oats or rolled
barley (not instant or quick-
cooking oats)
Natural muesli with no or few
cereal flakes in it (based
on oats, nuts, seeds and
dried fruit)
Extruded rice bran

grains—for boiling—to be
served with meals or added
to soups and salads

Barley—pearled, pot or
cracked
Basmati rice
Doongara rice
Wild rice
Quinoa
Whole buckwheat kernels
Burghul (cracked wheat)
Whole rye kernels

pasta and noodles

All types of durum wheat
pasta—fresh or dried; plain,
wholemeal or protein-
enriched
Ravioli, tortellini
Gluten-free split pea and soy
pasta
Dried mung bean noodles
(lungkow beanthread or
cellophane)
Fresh rice noodles
(not dried)
Soba (buckwheat) noodles

cookies

Cookies that contain lots of
dried fruit, whole rolled oats,
and stoneground flour

fruit

FRESH FRUIT
Apples, pears, oranges,
mandarins, tangerines,
grapefruit, plums, apricots,
nectarines, peaches, berries,
bananas (not over-ripe),
grapes, kiwi fruit, mango,
custard apple, avocado
(high-fat—eat in moderation)
DRIED FRUIT
Apple, apricot, pear, peach,
prunes, sultanas
CANNED FRUIT IN NATURAL
JUICE
peaches, pears
FRUIT JUICE—PURE,
UNSWEETENED, NO

ADDED SUGAR
Apple, grapefruit, orange,
pineapple, tomato

vegetables—fresh, canned
and frozen

Butternut pumpkin and all-
purpose (waxy) potatoes—
not mashed
Green peas
Carrots, carrot juice
Sweet corn
All non-starchy, low-carb
vegetables—onions, garlic,
shallots, leeks, herbs,
arugula, ginger, chilies,
tomatoes, lettuce, celery,
cucumber, cabbage,
mushrooms, brussels
sprouts, broccoli,
cauliflower, bell peppers,
spinach, green beans, snake
beans, kale, bean sprouts,
alfalfa, zucchini, eggplant,
artichokes, endive, chard,
swiss chard, bok choy and
other Asian greens, okra,
asparagus
Commercial tabouleh salad
(look for the least oily
looking ones)

legumes

All types of legumes—dried,
canned, vacuum packed (e.g.
lentils, chickpeas, soy beans,
kidney beans, cannellini
beans, four bean mix)

Reduced-fat hummus dip
Tofu
Tempeh
Canned baked beans

nuts and seeds

All types of raw or
dry-roasted nuts and seeds
—eat in moderation (Use
flax seeds, ground flax seed
meal, walnuts and pecans in
preference. These are
relatively good sources of
essential omega-3 fatty
acids, which many people
don't eat enough of.)

dairy products and some alternatives (fresh, frozen, long-life)

Cows' milk—full-fat,
reduced-fat and
low-fat; plain or flavored
Soy milk, calcium-enriched—
full-fat, reduced-fat, and
low-fat
Fermented milk drinks
Yogurt—all types
Custard
Ice cream—reduced and low-
fat
Pudding—made from instant
mix with milk
Mousse—made from instant
mix with milk or water; or
reduced-fat varieties in chilled
section of supermarket

Fromage frais products
All types of cheese—cottage,
ricotta, reduced-fat cheddar
and mozzarella

beverages

Bottled water—mineral,
spring, soda
Diet soft drinks and diet
cordials
Low-GI fruit juices
(fresh in fridge or
long-life)

sweeteners, condiments and other pantry staples

Sugar substitutes
Diet jams or pure fruit
spreads with no added
sugar
Yeast extract spreads
Low-fat mayonnaise
and diet salad
dressings
Vinegar, mustard, chili sauce,
mirin
Dried herbs and spices,
capers, fresh herb mixes for
fridge
Custard powder
Reduced-salt soy sauce
Canola and olive oil, canola
and olive oil spray,
reduced-fat canola
or olive oil margarine
Long-life lime juice and lemon
juice
Grated parmesan cheese

meat, poultry, fish and seafood—fresh, frozen, canned

Lean cuts of meat and lower-
fat premium ground meat
Poultry—fresh or frozen and
eaten without the skin
Eggs
Low-fat deli meats and
sausages
Fish—fresh or frozen;
canned in spring water or flavored in foil packages
Seafood—fresh, frozen
or canned
Sushi

soup—canned or dried

Minestrone

Lentil

Tomato

Clear beef, chicken or
vegetable

187

CONTACT INFORMATION FOR DIABETES SUPPORT GROUPS

USA—American Diabetes Association
1701 North Beauregard Street
Alexandria, VA 22311
Phone: 1 800 342 2383
Email: AskADA@diabetes.org
Web: www.diabetes.org

CANADA—Canadian Diabetes Association
National Life Building, 1400-522 University Ave
Toronto, ON M5G 2R5
Phone: 1 800 226 8464
Email:info@diabetes.ca
Web: www.diabetes.ca

AUSTRALIA—Diabetes Australia
5th Floor, 39 London Circuit
Canberra City, ACT 2600
Phone: 02 6232 3800
Email: admin@diabetesaustralia.com.au
Web: www.diabetesaustralia.com.au

INTERNATIONAL DIABETES INSTITUTE
250 Kooyong Road
Caulfield, Victoria 3162
Phone: 03 9258 5050
Email: admin@idi.org.au
Web: www.diabetes.com.au

NEW ZEALAND—Diabetes New Zealand National Office
PO BOX 12-1441, Thorndon, Wellington
Phone: 04 499 7145
Email: info@diabetes.org.nz
Web: www.diabetes.org.nz

UNITED KINGDOM—Diabetes UK
Macleod House
10 Parkway, London NW1 7AA
Phone: 020 7424 1000
Email: info@diabetes.org.uk
Web: www.diabetes.org.uk

INDEX